RELATIONAL
MEDICINE
*Perso*nalizing Modern Healthcare

The Practice of High-Tech Medicine as a Relational*Act*

RELATIONAL MEDICINE

*Person*alizing Modern Healthcare

The Practice of High-Tech Medicine as a Relational*Act*

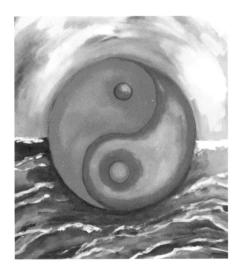

FEDERICA RAIA
MARIO DENG

University of California, Los Angeles, USA

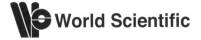 **World Scientific**

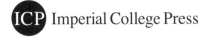 Imperial College Press

Published by

World Scientific Publishing Co. Pte. Ltd.
5 Toh Tuck Link, Singapore 596224
USA office: 27 Warren Street, Suite 401-402, Hackensack, NJ 07601
UK office: 57 Shelton Street, Covent Garden, London WC2H 9HE

Library of Congress Cataloging-in-Publication Data
Raia, Federica, author.
  Relational medicine : personalizing modern healthcare : the practice of high-tech medicine as a
RelationalAct / Federica Raia, Mario Deng.
    p. ; cm.
  Includes bibliographical references and index.
    ISBN 978-9814579681 (hardcover : alk. paper) -- ISBN 978-9814616300 (pbk. : alk. paper)
  I. Deng, Mario C., author. II. Title.
  [DNLM: 1. Heart Failure--psychology. 2. Biomedical Technology. 3. Cardiac Surgical
Procedures--psychology. 4. Personhood. 5. Physician-Patient Relations. WG 370]
  RC685.C53
  616.1'290651--dc23
                                                                          2014013669

British Library Cataloguing-in-Publication Data
A catalogue record for this book is available from the British Library.

In-house Editor: Darilyn Yap

Typeset by Stallion Press
Email: enquiries@stallionpress.com

Printed in Singapore by B & Jo Enterprise Pte Ltd

To our inspiring poets, the patients and their families
who have participated in this research project.

FOREWORD

Our vision at UCLA Health is "to heal humankind one patient at a time by improving health, alleviating suffering and delivering acts of kindness". And while *US News & World Report* ranks us the No. 5 hospital in the United States and, for more than 20 years, the "Best in the West", what makes us proudest is what our patients say about us. Our patient satisfaction scores are now among the best in the nation, and our transformation to a patient-centered model for excellence was described by author Joseph Michelli in his 2011 *New York Times* best-seller *Prescription for Excellence*.

If we were to change one word in our vision statement, it would be to replace *patient* with *person* — "to heal humankind one *person* at a time by improving health, alleviating suffering and delivering acts of kindness". Then we have the perfect starting point from which to embark on the journey that UCLA Professors Federica Raia and Mario Deng are inviting us upon in their fascinating and groundbreaking book *Relational Medicine: Personalizing Modern Healthcare — The Practice of High-Tech Medicine as a RelationalAct.*

What are the ingredients for a prescription for excellence that will improve health and alleviate suffering in this era of modern medicine in which organ transplantation and artificial organs are taken as a regular part of our lives? What is necessary to improve health and alleviate suffering one person at a time? The answer is straightforward: We need to think of the modern miracles of organ transplantation and artificial organs and personhood within one framework. When it comes to modern medicine, we cannot leave our personhood outside the hospital entrance.

As healthcare practitioners, we need to integrate organ transplantation and artificial organs and the basic human right of personhood into our daily professional experience. Only if healthcare professionals experience their own personhood in their daily practice can they convey the integration of personhood and body to their patients.

By practicing the Relational*Act*, healthcare providers can learn to achieve this goal.

David T. Feinberg, MD, MBA
President, UCLA Health System

ACKNOWLEDGMENTS

This book project is part of our Relational Medicine Project. We are indebted to all our patients and their families who made this project happen. For over more than a decade, invaluable inspiration and support came from our interaction with patients and their family members in New York City and Los Angeles.

An important early encounter was with Ms. Candace Moose and her husband Mr. James Moose in the fall of 2001 when she acutely fell ill with giant cell myocarditis and required urgent heart transplantation, sharing her experience in her book *The Grateful Heart — Diary of a Heart Transplant*. Subsequently, Candace and Jim, along with Mr. Robert Milo and his wife Mrs. Amy Milo, joined our invitation to become, together with Ms. Vanda Monaco-Westerstahl and Mr. John Henry Davis, founding members of the Relational Medicine Foundation (www.RelationalMedicineFoundation.org). The continued conversations with them, and subsequently also with Mr. Bruce Goldstein and Mr. James Billett laid the foundation for the encounter research that forms the basis of this book.

After our move from New York to Los Angeles, wholehearted support for the project came from Dr. David Feinberg, the CEO and President of the UCLA Health System, as well as from Dr. Eugene Washington, Dean of the David-Geffen School of Medicine at UCLA, Dr. Alan Fogelman, Executive Chair of the UCLA Department of Medicine, and Dr. James Weiss, Chief of the UCLA Division of Cardiology. At UCLA, Ms. Meredith Flynn joined the Relational Medicine Foundation and became an instrumental force in the critical advancement of the project. Among the growing number of UCLA patients, the artist Ms. Ann Donato stood out, as she inspired, after going through her own experience of left ventricular assist device implantation and subsequent heart transplantation, the book cover.

Federica's UCLA Relational*Act*Model (RAM) research lab would not have produced results if it had not been for the enthusiastic and critical participation of three cardiologists in Mario's UCLA Integrated Advanced Heart Failure/Mechanical Circulatory Support/Heart Transplantation Program, Dr. Martin Cadeiras, Dr. Daniel Cruz, and Dr. Ali Nsair, in the regular RAM-CoGen research sessions.

Invaluable research assistance and inspiration came from Federica's UCLA lab-students, Ms. Claire Alvarenga, Ms. Kristina Barrientos, Ms. Grecia Ramos, and Ms. Valeria M. Rivera.

We remember Ruggiero de Ritis, inspiring teacher and dear friend who awakened Federica as a young scholar into a new dialogic relation with continental philosophy. Seminars and activities at the Instituto Italiano per gli Studi Filosofi (Naples, Italy) with Ruggiero were always followed by critical and invaluable discussions in the best Italian intellectual tradition: while sharing a luscious meal and friendly wine.

Over the years of researching and writing this book, continued crucial inspirational feedback was provided by Mario's mother, Eva Deng, who rejuvenated with every step that the project matured.

CONTENTS

INTRODUCTION

It is often the custom to begin the introduction of a book by explaining how the idea of the book came about, what the book is about and conclude with how the book is organized. We altered this structure slightly; before we organize your reading of this book, we would like you to first follow us, albeit figuratively, on the Cardiothoracic Intensive Care Unit (CTICU) floor.

Medical Encounters in High-Tech Modern Medicine

Today I shadow the attending[1] advanced heart failure cardiologist, Dr. Mario Deng, on hospital medical rounds.

It is 6:30 AM and we have just entered the CTICU. I look around, trying to understand what it is that gives me the sense of openness here, but my attention is immediately captured by a group of health professionals congregated just outside a room, a patient's room. They are silently looking into the room. A physician comes toward us; my host Dr. Deng introduces me: "This is Prof. Raia," then turns to him to ask about updates. Dr. Vai is the advanced heart failure cardiology fellow,[1] a very dignified presence, he

---

[1]An attending is a physician on call responsible in her/his medical specialty for the hospitalized patients. Dr. Deng is a medical doctor who, after medical school, completed six years of internal medicine training, then specialized for three additional years in heart diseases. After these three years of general cardiology training (Cardiology Fellowship), he then specialized in advanced heart failure cardiology to take care of patients with advanced heart failure including those needing mechanical circulatory support and heart transplantation (Advanced Heart Failure and Transplant Cardiology fellowship). While this is a common training path for all cardiologists specializing in advanced heart failure, the years of training in the different specialization (e.g., cardiology fellowship, advanced heart failure and transplantation fellowship) varies by national training and specialization requirements. Because of the complexity of the heart failure syndrome, this specialization also requires broad knowledge in immunology, microbiology, and other related internal medicine disciplines.

stands tall and straight, his voice low and kind when updating the attending, my host Dr. Deng, on the emergency situation.

A patient is very sick. Mr. More. He is sedated.

Dr. Vai gives an almost imperceptible side shake to his head, moving his face in a grimace, his chin pushed up, the lips tighten with their corners pulled down expressing something like 'how sad' or 'I cannot believe it'.

We approach the room; the glass doors are completely opened. Five healthcare professionals are inside the room; others are coming and going. Some are discussing, looking at the patient, looking at the monitors, then back at the patient. Others are intervening on the patient with cuts, tubes sucking the blood, large clamps attached to his leg. It is an emergency. It is an emergency, yet the voices, the movements, rather than urgent, are precise, efficient, coordinated and all at low volume. It is as if all that really counts is concentrated in one small space, in a gaze, in a movement. There are questions on how it happened. I see it in the tense focused faces of the intensive care attending doctors and fellows, one just walking in the room with large dark circles under the wide-open, almost round, bloodshot eyes; I see it in the silence of the nurses. They are worried, they are astounded, they are mad, they are sad; it is grave but the volume is low. What a difference from the dramas I see on TV; the shouting, the running, the loud emotions thick as curtains. Here, it is grave but the volume is low.

The patient is intubated. Naked on the hospital bed. Catheters are cutting out of his flesh, from almost every part of his body: legs, arms, belly, chest, mouth. The intensive care bedside nurse and the cardiothoracic surgical fellow, wearing disposable yellow coats and blue thick gloves, are performing a surgical procedure, inserting and moving tubes in the patient's legs, in his groin. Their movements are precise, efficient, coordinated, not hectic; they must focus on stabilizing the patient. They are. They are focused on the organs failing, on blood clotting.

The patient is intubated, blood stains his naked body. Blood splatters over the nurse's and surgical fellow's disposable yellow coats, on their clogs, on the floor. All the attention focused on the bed scene: the surgeon and nurse working incessantly on the patient's body.

Healthcare professionals entering the room wear the yellow coat and the blue gloves. They stop a few steps away from the scene, forming a semicircle around the patient, the nurse, the surgical fellow. They look from monitors to patient, to surgeon, to nurse and back to monitors. They exchange brief comments, a few nods; indicate the blood collected in a transparent container, trends on the monitors and the patient's inert body.

Farther out, near the door, another group of healthcare professionals is watching the entire scene. They are closer to me and I can hear them discussing the case gently. What has happened? How exactly? What time did it start?

Next to me, just outside the room, in another semicircle formed around its entrance, another group. They also exchange a few comments, a few questions about the family, when to talk to them, what to say, "He was doing so well yesterday".

I am so impressed, almost to tears, seeing the care, all so gently, precisely, purposefully given; the faces of many look tired, worried, yet there is gentleness in the movement, in the voices. I can picture being at the outer circle of a giant spiral. Closest to the patient "the here and now": stabilizing the patient, now. As the spiral's sides open away from the bed, the space incorporates larger dimensions; the time scale opens to a trajectory: how the patient had been responding in the last hour. Farther away on a par with the distance from the patient's bed, the time scale expands to reach the past 24 hours. The last, in furthermost position from the patient's bed in the concentric semicircles of health professionals, as to incorporate all, the entire life trajectory including the patient's future and his family. Here I can feel their worries, their bewilderment, their sadness, their pain.

The impression is of a place where blood, breathing, suffering, dying, living all have their own space, each with multiple layers of being in existence, the gene, the molecule, the tissue, the organ, the person, all have their own dignity.

Doctors in medical encounters zoom in, from the encounter with another person, the patient — hello, how are you? — down to the organs, the tissues, to the molecular, to the gene level and zoom back out from the microscopic world to tissue, organ, phenotype, to the person level; they do it in one movement, one single necessarily uninterrupted movement for making decisions about diagnoses, treatment options, and how to live with them, in the *here and now* at the person level.

In the CTICU, the organized distribution in different discourse levels around the patient's bed allows focusing: on the organ, on the recent medical course, on life and death, on the person level, Mr. More's life.

'We need to . . .'

The advanced heart failure cardiologist's voice, my host's voice, calls me back. What? In that moment, I realize he is one of the doctors wearing the yellow coat and blue gloves, attending to the patient.

'We need to talk to the family. We will be back . . . they don't need us here now. Later, when they are done . . .'

'Hello Mrs. More.'

She is expecting news. She leaves the chair in the small private waiting room where she has been waiting since last night when her husband, recovering from LVAD[2] implantation, suddenly developed ventricular fibrillation. He needed to be resuscitated. An emergency surgery was performed to implant another device, a short-term mechanical assist device to help his heart pump more oxygenated blood through the body. But Mr. More had started bleeding internally.

'Hello Dr. Deng.'

He takes her hand and keeps it in his own until she sits again. He sits in the only empty chair left, just in front of her chair. In the waiting room, six other people are sitting, family members. On her left, her son, a young man. He looks speechless, staring at the floor. Next to him, a young woman looking at the doctor. An older man, Mrs. More's brother, sits on her other side with his wife and another woman is sitting next to the doctor. The cardiology fellow, three students and I gather around the open door, the room is too small to accommodate all of us.

'You have my contact, my card with all the numbers, the cellphone, the pager. You can get in touch with me anytime, you know.'

She knows.

Silence.

He has spoken so slowly that I can write every word he says.

The doctor looks at the rest of the family and looks back to Mrs. More.

---

[2] As will be detailed in Chapter 1, a Left Ventricular Assist Device (LVAD) is a mechanical pump that pumps or helps to pump blood from the left ventricle of the heart to the rest of the body.

'The last twelve hours were not good.'

Silence.

Dr. Deng waits until she nods.

'Overnight he had a fast heartbeat and he was also bleeding so the heart function is not the way it should be.'

She nods, he continues.

'That is why he needed the short-term assist heart pump and now ... with all that he is still bleeding.'

Silence.

She nods.

'That is not a good situation,' he continues, looking at Mrs. More. 'The bleeding is having effects on the liver, on the kidney.' He talks in simple sentences, slowly, as if the words are originating from the silence in the room, his long pauses making it dense.

Silence.

Mrs. More looks at him.

Dr. Deng recounts how well Mr. More was recovering; yes, she nods.

'... and this is unexpected,' he continues. Slowly. 'I wanted to update you and we will continue to do so on how he is doing.'

'How was the conversation last night with Dr. Ashir?' Mrs. More recounts the meeting with the surgeon during the early morning hours after Dr. Ashir was called in for the emergency surgery for the short-term pump implantation in Mr. More's chest.

Dr. Deng listens to her very attentively. She knows there are uncertainties. It could go either way. He could get worse but he could recover. She has hope.

Dr. Deng does not remove his gaze from her and with the same kindness, the same slow pace, he starts revisiting what has happened. Every word is a new step; a fundamental pillar of understanding of what life is about. The same occurrences, but now he introduces stronger words in his sentences: what before was 'unexpected' becomes 'very unfortunate' and I understand. He wants to know where she is. She has hope. Now he is moving her to prepare for an understanding and acceptance of the possibility of death.

He does it slowly with much care, waiting for her to allow him to continue. All these silences, pauses. I can think of a scene where a parent encourages a toddler to take a step, one step and a second and a third, slowly, allowing the baby more and more space to try further consecutive steps. She does, feeling safe, she toddles toward the adult and passes the parent; she is on her own, she can walk on her own. There, a moving into life, here in the CTICU, moving toward another part of life: death.

Mrs. More has been slowly nodding, looking at Dr. Deng:

'What do you think of the situation?'

Dr. Deng revisits the medical situation; again, adding more details and repeating others, they are now sinking deeper.

Then: 'So ...'

The approximately eight-second-long silence is communicating as much as the words. She nods, he continues:

'While all that is going on now is continuing,

(a silence, about three seconds)

chances for a good outcome are diminishing ...'

Long, long, long silence. I count 20 seconds.

Dr. Deng does not remove his gaze from Mrs. More.

She turns to the other family members and asks if they have anything to ask. At this point, the doctor repeats that she has all his contact numbers including the cellphone and gives her his card, again: 'You can call me anytime. We will be back, but at any time you want to have an update ...'

'This is an ongoing emergency situation ...'

He does not move, he is sitting in front of her. No sign of leaving, instead he asks her impression of Mr. More's health during the last day. She is not sure; he was doing well, but something was a little off. She could not say what precisely, he just looked a little off.

Mrs. More and Dr. Deng talk about Mr. More's entire medical course up until the previous night, then Dr. Deng continues the narrative on what happened during the past hours, again, now adding more details, his words sink even deeper if ever possible.

And again: 'It is unfortunate.'

He stops.

'What is your suggestion?' Mrs. More asks.

'I want you to know this,' he pauses.

'You are his decision maker.'

His gaze, always on her. She starts crying silently.

The doctor is leaning toward her and she toward him.

All the others are silent.

She slowly nods.

The doctor continues, it is time to tell, she is ready to hear: there is a possibility that at some point somebody from the team will come out to ask her what her decision is.

She is silently crying. Not the only one.

'I want you and the family to be together and talk.'

All in the room including us listening in at the door are brought to the same point: death is imminent. Death as part of life.

The doctor stands up and embraces Mrs. More.

We leave.

The encounter is over.

I feel slow; I feel I don't have enough weight, I am not thick enough, too vacuous to walk.

I look at the students rounding with us and I see I am not alone.

We left our body weight in that room.

We go back to Mr. More's room. Many health professionals, some are inside the room, others are coming and going. Not a good sign, I learn. Mr. More is still intubated; naked on the bed. Catheters are coming out of almost each part of his body: legs, arms, belly, chest, mouth. The CTICU nurse and cardiothoracic surgical fellow have just terminated the surgical procedure. The patient lies immobile, his penis lies on his leg in a deathly sleep. I think he would not want me to look at him like this. I move, but there is no need. The cardiothoracic surgical fellow gently covers Mr. More's lower body. They had to insert tubes in the legs, in the groin, but, now, there is no need for this nakedness, this bare body. The patient is a *person*.

'I talked to the family,' Dr. Deng says.

Many look at him. The critical care attending who had just walked out of the room to talk to Dr. Deng looks at him, his shoulders lower, deflate, in a sense of relief: 'Thank you.'

They are trying to stabilize the patient at least for the bleeding; the critical care physician shakes his head, a sorrowful expression on his face. It is good that somebody has talked to the family, another complex moment in itself.

'We need to continue. We will be back.'

What?

'We need to continue the rounds on the other patients. We will be back … they don't need us here now. Later …'

Once again Dr. Deng's voice calls me back.

I follow him next door. Another center, another patient, another *person*, another life full of stories, experiences, loved ones, fears, memories, fights, losses, victories.

We enter.

About This Book

It is with the advanced heart failure medical encounter of Mrs. and Mr. More that we ask you to start reading this book, without *a priori* explanation and clarification of how the book is organized. While this entrance facilitates introducing ourselves as practitioner and researcher in our practice contexts and with our respective standpoints, it also offers a glimpse into the human experiences as we discuss them in this book.

Mrs. and Mr. More's experience of encountering death as part of life is a person-level experience, just as it is a person-level experience for someone being kept alive mechanically by a machine that is assisting or in some cases replacing the person's heart as this person continues to participate in ordinary family, work and social life. Interaction with and integration of such high-technology medicine into a person's life constitute the experiences of patients with advanced heart failure and their families, as well as the experiences of the healthcare professionals taking care of them. Unthinkable 30 years ago, these experiences, of the person in interaction with high-tech modern medicine, are novel to patients and their family caregivers and unknown to healthcare professionals.

In this book, we explore the process of practicing high-tech modern medicine in advanced heart failure as a process where integration of science, technology and personhood in the medical encounter emerges.

From the biomedical perspective, the course of this disease is unpredictable, the prognosis uncertain and the therapeutic options continuously evolve with scientific and technological advances.

Advanced heart failure practice, with its novel and unknown experiences of the person in interaction with the technological advancements of modern medicine and its uncertainties at the biomedical/clinical level, is a practice 'in the making'. Bruno Latour (1987), studying the processes of creating scientific knowledge in the natural sciences, describes this process as having two faces like the mythological figure of the Roman god *Janus bifrons*. In Roman mythology, Janus' two faces are gazing in opposite directions. One, gazing into the past, faces what has ended, what is known. The other, gazing into the future, faces the unknown. Latour, by studying the emergence of scientific knowledge, considers it a process 'in the making' monitored by Janus's gaze into what is becoming, what is questioned. By taking this approach, Latour unveils the importance of the social dimension in the scientific knowledge-forming process.

Advanced heart failure practice has the quality of being 'in the making' not only from the characteristics of uncertainty and novelty due to the continuous evolution of medical knowledge and the technological advancement in the last 30 years, but also because it is unfolding in the interactions of persons with different knowledge, understandings and perceptions of the manifestation of the disease.

It is in the practice of medicine, in the interaction between healthcare professionals, patients and their families that it is possible to observe how knowledge, understanding, acceptance of advanced heart failure high-tech medicine is discussed, shared, modified and utilized to become integrated into people's lives. Integration of science, technology and personhood is a process in the *practice* of high-tech modern medicine. This practice is the departure point and the returning point of this book.

In the following section on our method, we describe how we study this practice which we believe cannot be approached and classified from the individual perspectives on the illness, on the disease, on the medical science and on the use of technology. We describe the research model we developed to study the advanced heart failure practice as proceeding *iteratively* in three stages of data collection and analysis; as a learning model, each stage is necessary to generate resources for the other stages to emerge and develop. In this section, we also describe how our collaboration unfolds as it has brought us to the understanding of the advanced heart failure practice that would never have emerged if we had worked in isolation: a researcher alone, a doctor alone, without the other. This understanding permeates the entire book. As it is often the case when working with someone from another field of research, bringing perspectives together ensures that they will look different, maybe messier but nevertheless richer in their interconnectedness.

In Chapter 1, we set the premises from which we start. Here we introduce and start bringing together the disease, the illness experiences and the medical and technological advances in advanced heart failure from their original separate domains of investigation. We utilize the poetry of the medieval Italian poet, Dante Alighieri, to help us resonate with the experiences in a health crisis of advanced heart failure, and the existential phenomenological perspective of the German philosopher Martin Heidegger, to help us make sense of the person's experience in the practice of high-tech modern medicine.

In Chapter 2, with the help of video- and audio-recordings of their in-patient medical encounters, we enter the medical practice of advanced heart failure and accompany patient, family and doctor in their in-patient encounters. We analyze and discuss the complexity of these encounters emerging from the process of integration of personhood, science and technology and we identify the recurrent aspects of these medical encounters in high-tech modern medicine.

In Chapter 3, while continuing to follow patient, family and doctor in their in-patient medical encounters, we identify four different phases common to each of these encounters: preparation, initiation, continuation and conclusion. We discuss how each of these phases varies in response to the encounter situation in the specificity of the disease and the needs of the persons involved. Here, bringing together discussions from previous chapters, we begin to define what we call the Relational*Act* encounter in high-tech modern medicine.

In Chapter 4, we follow patients and their families and doctors in their in-patient medical encounters. We explore different practice patterns as seen at different levels of mastering medical practice (Dreyfus & Dreyfus, 2000). We discuss the concept of the Relational*Act* dyad in medical practice and its relevance in the different scenarios and practices of taking care of the person in advanced heart failure. Here we discuss the process of learning to integrate science, technology and personhood in high-tech modern medicine from the perspective of the doctors.

In Chapter 5, we follow a heart transplant patient into the *out*patient clinic. We describe the medical practice using the classical diagnostic tools to monitor heart transplantation rejection based on organ pathology — the heart muscle biopsy. We compare it with the medical practice based on modern high-technology and scientific research, the method of a genomic biomarker blood test, and its effect on personalizing patient care.

Chapter 6 concludes the book with reflections on concepts and theories of medicine that have helped shaped our Relational Medicine research, concept and practice.

Method

Formulating the question

The study of the *practice* of high-tech modern medicine as it is in advanced heart failure can be a daunting task. Where do we start? We are interested in the *relational* aspect of the medical encounter, and specifically how the *interactions* among stakeholders (e.g., patients, family, healthcare professionals) with different knowledge, experiences, understandings and perceptions of the manifestation of the disease shape integration of science, technology and personhood in the medical practice of high-tech modern medicine.

As in the case of Mrs. and Mr. More, CTICU interactions among stakeholders are many and differentiated. Do we study the interactions of all health professionals in the advanced heart failure team with patients and with families? They are all important. How about the interactions among healthcare professionals? Oh yes, also important. Where do we study them, in meetings where decisions must be made for transplant evaluation, during rounds in the hospital as we saw the complexity unfolding in the CTICU, in research labs? What do we study about the interactions? Communication? About what? Laboratory analysis prescribed? Yes. Laboratory results? Yes. Medical notes? Yes. All are important to help characterize a practice, as Annemarie Mol shows in her ethnographic work of atherosclerosis (2002), and important to characterize the multi-level complexity of advanced heart failure practice.

Should we collect all of the above, or do we restrict our research to those objects, medical tools, communications, that enter into interactional situations of a medical encounter? Which technological integration do we choose, and when do we study the interactions with these biomedical technologies: before surgery, after surgery, when decisions need to be made, or do we study the interactions with these biomedical technologies during longer intervals of time? These are important methodological questions because, as we have noted above and describe in detail in the book, there is no linear stage-like progression in advanced heart failure. For example, patients who had a mechanical circulatory support device implantation as bridge to transplantation, can, after heart transplantation, undergo another mechanical circulatory support device implantation or an implantation of a cardioverter-defibrillator or a second heart transplantation.

For how long do we study the practice of advanced heart failure in medical encounters, one day, two days, a week, a year? That is, do we sample a few encounters per patient and have many patients in the study, or do we follow fewer patients and healthcare professionals, but follow their medical encounters over time? The first approach presupposes that medical encounters in advanced heart failure do not change over time and that the experiences of all patients at any time are similar enough that aggregating them would give a reasonably complete sample to work with. The second approach questions this assumption and opens up new questions regarding generalizability of results.

In reading about Mr. and Mrs. More's story, the reader could have made a longer list of questions regarding people, places, rooms, biomedical objects and tools, actions, symbols, that needed to be considered in exploring advanced heart failure practice.

Wherever and however we start, we find ourselves always in the midst of things, of people's lives, of people's stories, of career paths, of technological advancements, of disease paths, of illness experiences, of hospital rooms, of laboratory work, and of research labs' lives (Latour & Woolgar, 1986).

In following Dr. Deng, encountering Mrs. More, one realizes that in their communication, while there are references to organs, machines, tools and procedures, nothing points towards the specific content that would indicate that Dr. Deng is preparing Mrs. More to encounter death as part of life. One finds nothing that can be extracted as a general principle of communication of death as part of life. Even though organs, machines, tools and procedures are part of the medical talk as are silences, nods, and repetition of content, nothing explains how one finds him/herself, as all participants in that encounter do, in the transition into making sense of the 'possibility of the impossibility of any existence at all" (Heidegger, 1927/1962, p. 262/307). One finds nothing pointing towards a rational/discrete approach on how to communicate death as part of life and nothing pointing towards an isolable rule or moment when Dr. Deng and Mrs. More both know they understand, one that the Other is ready to accept death, the Other accepting it. Nothing.

So our question is: how is this *nothing*?

To address this question, we enter this complex and rich field following one person, Dr. Deng, whose perspective is, to start with, deeply rooted and immersed in the practice of advanced heart failure care as he has been practicing in this field for more than 25 years. His way of practicing medicine, his way of dealing with each specific situation, each as complex as it can be as we witnessed in the CTICU, does not follow *a priori* rules. Dr. Deng, in his encounter with Mrs. More, enacts what we perceived and called the *nothing*, as it cannot be reduced to application of predefined abstract principles. In Pierre Bourdieu's terms (Bourdieu, 1977), Dr. Deng has a "sense of the game", a know-how that a beginner or even competent practitioner does not have yet: he knows his practice better than any general rules or principles can describe (King, 2000). His mastering of the practice (Dreyfus & Dreyfus, 2000), as it is enacted in tailoring it to each specific situation, is considered appropriate and proper by others in the situational context: patients and their family, nurses and other physicians. As shown in the encounter with Mrs. More, Dr. Deng's relational actions (talking, gesturing, entering a room, etc.) not only respond to the specific situation in his own unique way, but also help the participants in that specific situation change their perception of the situation.

It is by studying his medical practice in advanced heart failure that we develop a sense, informed by a practitioner's understanding, of what the high-tech medicine practice in advanced heart failure can look like.

Collaborating

In 2009, we started a series of informal conversations around issues of scientific and technological advancement in persons' lives as seen in advanced heart failure. These conversations were followed by exploratory interviews in which Mario (Dr. Deng) as practitioner and his patients and their families narrate their experiences in advanced heart failure.

We (Federica and Mario) initiated our collaboration as a participatory research project, involving the practitioners (i.e., Mario) in the research process from the initial stages as co-researchers. From our perspectives and interests, as scientists and as educators, participatory research is a powerful research approach because along with those who study the practices from the 'outside' (researchers, i.e., Federica), those whose practice is studied (doctors, i.e., Mario) also learn from the research.

Learning about one's own practice, reflecting on it in collaboration with other practitioners ('insiders') and researchers ('outsiders') can be potentially transformative for practitioners' own practices of medicine (i.e., Mario's practice) and transformative for the training of medical professionals.

Participatory research is also an important experience for the researcher (i.e., Federica) because it moves the research in directions enriched by questions most relevant to practice and anchors it in what is relevant to stakeholders. In addition, it requires the researcher (Federica) to learn about advanced heart failure as a disease, to read related textbooks and journal publications, to attend international and national heart failure conferences and follow hospital rounds.

We chose the approach of participatory research because the richness of the medical encounters in high-tech modern medicine cannot be unveiled by a single perspective of either the (outsider) researcher or the (insider) practitioner alone. This is because there are interactions among persons (patient, healthcare professional, family caregiver), each with their complementary role and perspective in the encounter. There is knowledge about one's body (patient) and knowledge of the body of the Other (healthcare professional, family caregiver) that changes; there is knowledge of science and technology and its integration in the medical encounter, and there are the experiences of illness, disease and care.

In working from our different and complementary perspectives, we strive to understand how different levels — the biological, the social and the medical — shape the medical encounters in high-tech modern medicine.

Studying the practice

To study this practice of high-tech modern medicine, we developed a research model that proceeds *iteratively* in three stages of data collection and

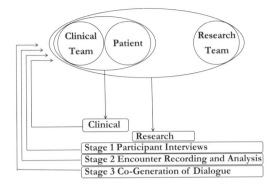

Figure M.1: Relational*Act* Model (RAM): Iterative development of research in 3 stages (details see text).

analysis (Figure M.1). Each stage of the process with continuity of representation generates resources and structures necessary for the following stages to emerge. For example, the interviews provided an appreciation for how high-tech modern medicine experiences were recounted by stakeholders. Insights from Stages 2 and 3 (as described below) were utilized to shape subsequent interviews. The process served also as a validation process, because participants must recognize the practice patterns as authentic. It is a rich process that can transform practice and the understanding of it.

Participants

In addition to one of the authors, advanced heart failure physician Dr. Mario Deng, the healthcare professionals (i.e., physicians and nurses) from the hospital's advanced heart failure program, consented to participate in the study. Twenty-five patients and respective family caregivers were recruited as participants for this project. All participant patients, caregivers and physicians consenting to be part of the project were invited onto the research team. While three recruited physicians participated in weekly co-generative research meetings, the constraints of health conditions and time commitment impeded participation for patients and family caregivers interested in the weekly research meetings.

Except for the authors, the names of patients and their family and healthcare professionals reported here are pseudonyms. Dr. Deng will be called Dr. D from Chapter 1 when in interaction with patients. There are two reasons for this choice. The first is to remove the need to use 'his (mine)' when referring to Dr. Deng's perspectives (i.e., both in third and first person), making the book difficult to read. The second reason is the understanding that while it is Dr. D's practice we study here, there can be possible overlap and similarity with other physicians, as we discussed in the research meetings.

Data collection and analysis

We collected our data as part of an ethnographic and participatory research project (2009–2013) conducted in large university medical centers in New York and Los Angeles in three stages.

Field notes

Throughout the duration of the project, Federica took field notes when on medical rounds and when encountering participants outside the context of the formal interviews in the hospital. These notes are reported here as integrated in the text and with single quotation marks (i.e., 'quoted notes text' when a direct quote is given. Mr. and Mrs. More's encounter is based on such field notes.

Stage 1: *Narratives*. We conducted one- to two-hour-long interviews with participating patients and their families to collect their narratives on their experiences in advanced heart failure. The interviews were open-ended and flexible for questions that developed during the course of the interview, based on the interviewee's responses. This method of interviewing has been used in medical sociology (see Pierret, 2003; and Rier, 2010 for reviews) because it gives respondents time and opportunities to develop their answers and explore their beliefs and opinions without the limitation of pre-set questions, allowing patients and their family to report their own stories. These interviews were transcribed and analyzed for themes. Excerpts from the transcripts are reported here in double quotation marks "quoted interview text" and smaller font.

Stage 2: *Medical encounter recordings*. Depending on the setting, participating advanced heart failure cardiologists were audio- and video-recorded in their medical encounters with their patients. During *in*patient medical rounds only audio-recordings were made. In *out*patient clinic, both audio- and video-recordings were made of the medical encounters.

For medical encounters during *in*patient rounds, advanced heart failure cardiologists were audio-recorded while on rounds in the hospital with patients who were hospitalized for advanced heart failure. Such patients are often admitted or transferred from a regional hospital into the larger hospital in an advanced decompensated and often life-threatening condition. It is during these hospital rounds that advanced heart failure cardiologists meet the patients and their caregiver(s), often for the first time. It is during the stay in the hospital that patients and caregivers are (often) faced with fundamental decision-making challenges and situations as in Mr. and Mrs. More's case.

Each patient is in a single-bed room. In the Cardiothoracic Intensive Care Unit (CTICU), patients are recovering from cardiothoracic surgery, for example from a mechanical circulatory support device implantation or heart transplantation; in the Coronary Care Unit (CCU) and the Cardiac Observation Unit (COU) patients are under observation and often awaiting heart transplantation, with their names registered on the United Network for Organ Sharing (UNOS) waiting list. *In*patient medical rounds are structured so that the attending advanced heart failure cardiologist, the physician on call responsible for the hospitalized patients, walks from unit to unit, visiting each patient in her/his hospital room. The attending cardiologist rounds on 20–40 patients each day of the service.

Due to this structure, it is very difficult to videotape the encounters without interfering with the progression of the encounter and the medical rounds, nevertheless, the audio data itself offers a rare opportunity to study how a relationship between patient/caregiver and doctor is developing daily over a period of one or more weeks. Specifically, in one of the institutions, in an effort to maintain more continuity of care and less possibility of errors in transmission of information from one attending to the other, the advanced heart failure group organized the teaching[3] rounds so that one advanced heart failure attending cardiologist is on

---

[3] *Rounds* in university hospitals are also called *teaching rounds* as the teaching/learning component of the practice of medicine in which medical students, interns and residents, fellows, and attendings participate, is constitutive of the rounds.

service for two consecutive weeks including weekends. In other programs around the USA, the advanced heart failure service may be divided into slots of one week excluding the weekend (i.e., five days), splitting a two-week period service among four different advanced heart failure attending physicians.

In *out*patient clinic medical encounters, patients suffering from advanced heart failure are no longer hospitalized or not yet hospitalized. They come into the hospital for a medical appointment and meet with the advanced heart failure nurse and cardiologist in examination rooms. Patients, caregivers and health professional often refer to these hospital *out*patient visits as 'clinic' (visits).

Of the 25 patients in the study, 18 patients and their family were recorded in their medical encounters with the participating physician for a period of 1–2 years. These include both *in*patient and *out*patient visits. Their encounters were transcribed and analyzed for patterns. They are reported here in the transcribed form in smaller font: indicating the line of transcription, the speaker (e.g., Dr. D) and the spoken words:

15   Dr. D: Beautiful!

Stage 3: *Co-generative dialoguing (CoGen)*.[4] Advanced heart failure cardiologists, whose interactions have been recorded in Stage 2, participate weekly in two-hour-long audio/video-recording viewing sessions as part

---

[4]Elden & Levin (1991) conceptualized co-generative dialogue as a space where the diverse ways of understanding of the worker (insider) and the researcher (outsider) meet and where 'richness and quality of the research depends on the ability of the insiders and outsiders to play their different frameworks and expertise against each other to create a new, third explanatory framework'. Roth and Tobin (2004) further elaborate co-generative dialogue in contexts where researchers are also involved in the practice they are studying. For example, they study a co-teaching model in which one or more student teachers taught urban classes together, with a teacher, a university supervisor or researcher, or a school administrator. Class participants then participated in co-generative dialoguing sessions. In their work they find that "co-generative dialoguing really has become a praxis of method in a triple sense. First, it constitutes a concrete situation in which to generate theory as part of research. Second, it constitutes an alternative to interviewing teachers about their experiences; that is, we generated data first by co-teaching and then together by discursively evolving understandings of what happened. Third, and perhaps most importantly, it has become a means for all stakeholders in a situation to deal with contradiction and conflict and to design changes themselves rather than waiting for policies and recommendations from researchers" (p. 13).

of the research team. These research encounters are audio/videotaped. In these two-hour-long weekly sessions, the participating advanced heart failure cardiologists, together with the researchers, review the taped medical encounters in which they participated and discuss the elements that emerged. Everyone contributes to the discussion, sharing impressions of what has taken place. The point here, as Timmermans and Haas (2008) argue, is not "to extol the therapeutic successes and legitimize the power of physicians' authority" (p. 671). Rather, it is to explore how authority is used for healing or with the intent to heal, in a practice where, as we discuss in Chapter 1, integration of science, technology and personhood is required and where the experiences of high-tech modern advanced heart failure medicine, unthinkable 30 years ago, are novel to patients and their family caregivers and unknown to physicians.

Jointly reviewing the data in CoGen sessions allowed a richer perspective on the *practice* of high-tech modern advanced heart failure medicine to unfold and questions most relevant to practice to be addressed. These depend on the clinical circumstances and on the physician's stance and knowledge at specific times in the medical encounters (Wirtz, Cribb, & Barber, 2006).

It also allowed checking for validity of the emerging patterns identified in this study, as did our long and rich discussions during the last three years with two patients and their families in reviewing part of the data and its analysis. The CoGen sessions are analyzed for emerging patterns and themes. The results are discussed with the participants and the encounter recording is reviewed in the light of Stage 3 and Stage 1 insights.

Data from Stages 1 and 2 were transcribed. Three different people checked for any discrepancy of the transcriptions that were then reviewed and resolved during research meetings. Transcribed quotes from CoGen are reported in the main text and in double quotation marks: "transcribed CoGen quoted text".

When listening to the taped recordings of the medical encounters (recorded in Stage 2), we noticed long silences in Dr. D's medical interactions, similar to those occurring in the encounter with Mrs. More. A comparison of video- and audio-recorded medical encounters showed that except when a physical examination is being performed, these silences constitute a pattern of communication in Dr. D's medical encounters. When the silences occur after a patient has spoken, Dr. D has usually been either listening with his eyes closed or has been gazing at the person speaking for the entire time. Dr. D's conversation pattern in CoGen meetings does not show the same pattern of silences that we observed in the medical interactions. Based on this, we consider the silences to be specific to the medical interaction communication.

We analyzed the data from Stage 2 for the pattern of silences. We report silences that are longer than 900 milliseconds (0.9 seconds) as long silences are reported to cluster around the one-second interval (0.9–1.2 s) (Jefferson, 1989). They are indicated in parenthesis (0.9 s) and interpreted within the specific context in which they occur, that is, their meaning is attributed based on the location in the conversation, its surrounding talk and compared with the speaker's interpretation of the silence in CoGen meetings.

In Stage 2 data, we noticed patterns of overlapping talk, that is Dr. D and a patient occasionally talk at the same time. It is not a common pattern and when it emerges we report it in the transcripts. We use the following notation in the transcripts to make our interpretation of the medical talk clearer:

[word]
[word]

with words enclosed in square brackets aligned one beneath the other to denote the start and the end of overlapping talk as it is customary for adjacent lines in conversation analysis (Heritage & Maynard, 2006).

We also used the notation '::' to indicate that the speaker has stretched the preceding sound, for example in 'bu::t', the really stretched sound of the 'u' makes the word feels less definitive. So hearing 'bu::t' as compared to 'but' gives a completely different sense of what the speaker is uttering.

CHAPTER 1
STATUS QUO

What does it mean to address the status quo? One might think that in this chapter we could build on the rich literature of patient-doctor encounters in general/primary care and refer to the extensive literature documenting concerns with medical practice as patients' roles in their care change. We do not. We continue our exploration maintaining the focus on high-tech modern medicine. With the virtual absence of attention to high-tech medicine in chronic and acute advanced heart failure practice, often in the setting of critical care medicine, we need to come to a definition of what a status quo in high-tech modern medical practice really means.

Let us start by entering a consultation room during an advanced heart failure medical encounter.

We see three or even four people.

They are sitting.

One, sitting on a consultation bed, naked from the waist up, talks facing another person who is wearing a white coat; a third person dressed in a blue sweater sits next to ... Oh wait! The person sitting on the consultation bed has bandages on his abdomen and a tube is coming out of his belly through the bandages. It snakes from the bandages into a bag, to finally connect to a computerized system: "click clack, click clack, click clack", a mechanical sound is coming from the bag and ... oh! ... at the same time from the person's chest. In a hospital *out*patient examination room, during 'VAD clinic', the medical clinic for patients who have an implanted mechanical circulatory support device, three persons are talking; one, in the white coat, is an advanced heart failure cardiologist, one sitting high on the examination bed connected to a portable machine is a patient with advanced heart failure, "click clack, click clack, click clack", his mechanical circulatory support device is beating with the rhythm of a human heart; a third person, sitting in one of the two chairs next to the examination table, is a family caregiver. Can you imagine the topic of the conversation?

'I took a shower!'

Yes, in an advanced heart failure medical encounter, a patient living with an artificial heart, the advanced heart failure doctor and a family caregiver are talking about taking a shower. 'Not an easy thing to do,' the family caregiver is saying. 'We tried different possible ways to keep the water out of the driveline so the electrical motor would not short-circuit and stop. Not good!' No, not at all having the beloved die like that.

The patient smiles. 'After much trial and error … I took a shower! A twenty-minute-long shower!'

'Beautiful!' says the doctor.

They say their favorite opera is opening the next day. They look at the machine … click clack, click clack, click clack … in the silence of the theater. Will they go?

How to make sense of this scene?

Is it an issue of high technology in interaction with human life and how to design it in order to mesh them more efficiently so that Mr. Rice can take a shower without concerns? Is it an issue regarding a family caregiver scared of harming the loved one when helping him take a shower? Does the caregiver need more training? Or maybe it is an issue of structure of support? Is it a learning and cognitive issue of how to take a shower without dying as a result? Is it the experience of having one's body kept alive by a machine? Is it a medical issue of the body being able to survive outside an isolated sterilized environment? Is it the experience of the self, having an artificial heart completely substituting for one's own? Whose experience is this? The patient's, the doctor's, the family caregiver's? Some would say we are asking questions in the dualistic omnipresent problem of essence (i.e., matter, body) vs. existence (i.e., self, mind). This is not necessarily a framework we want to use. So we start by asking why the doctor responds to the simple act of taking a shower by saying, 'Beautiful!' What is beautiful here?

Starting from trying to make sense of the response 'beautiful' in relation to the patient and family caregiver experiences of taking a shower, we realize we need to know more about the circumstances, the context, the people involved, their story, how their interactions evolve, how they get to know each other and about each other, so as to share the meaning 'beautiful' in describing the taking of a shower, a strange comment for somebody from the outside.

So where to start addressing the status quo?

Wherever we start, there will be always somebody and something to relate to, to know, something before and something afterwards that needs to be part of our story to make sense of the experience, as we ourselves discovered when opening that door on an advanced heart failure medical encounter: *in medias res:* 'into the midst of things'.

Nel mezzo del cammin di nostra vita	Midway through the journey of our life, I found
mi ritrovai per una selva oscura,	myself in a dark wood, for I had strayed
ché la diritta via era smarrita.	3 from the straight pathway to this tangled ground.[1]

We start *in medias res* (*Nel mezzo del cammin di nostra vita*) at a point from where it is impossible to continue on the same path we were on; a turning point (Harrison, 1992).

We proceed in this chapter by presenting the complex human experience of illness, of disease and of the technological advances introduced in the medical practice in advanced heart failure. A practice that the three persons in the examination room are learning to handle, deal and cope with. We proceed, guided by the first Canto of Dante Alighieri's Divine Comedy. We chose this entrance because we feel that poetry, and Dante's Canto I in particular as the prelude to Dante's journey through Hell, Purgatory and Paradise, resonates with the human experience (*nostra vita/*our life) while recruiting the physicality of our body experiences as constitutive of the person's life journey. We call upon the Poet to help us recruit illness, disease and high-technology medicine as a human experience, because a person ultimately cannot experience them each in isolation. So, let us follow Dante until our paths diverge, he, going through Hell where there is individuality and isolation, desire and not hope;[2] we, entering the advanced heart failure medical practice where we find death as part of life, hope, transformation, care.

Nel mezzo del cammin di nostra vita	Midway through the journey of our life, I found
mi ritrovai per una selva oscura,	myself in a dark wood, for I had strayed
ché la diritta via era smarrita.	3 from the straight pathway to this tangled ground.

---

[1] English text source: The Divine Comedy of Dante Alighieri translated by Michael Palma (2008). *Inferno : A New Verse Translation, Backgrounds and Contexts, Criticism.* Giuseppe Mazzotta (Ed.). New York: W.W. Norton.

Italian text source: Project Gutenberg's The Project Gutenberg Etext "Divina Commedia di Dante: Inferno" In Italian with accents [8-bit text]. *This eBook is for the use of anyone anywhere at no cost and with almost no restrictions whatsoever. You may copy it, give it away or re-use it under the terms of the Project Gutenberg License included with this eBook or online at www.gutenberg.org.*

[2] *Inferno,* Canto IV, v. 43: "Che sanza speme vivemo in disio". *Purgatorio,* Canto XXIII, v. 2 and 23.

Ahi quanto a dir qual era è cosa dura	How hard it is to tell of, overlaid
esta selva selvaggia e aspra e forte	with harsh and savage growth, so wild and raw
che nel pensier rinova la paura!	6 the thought of it still makes me feel afraid.
Tant' è amara che poco è più morte;	Death scarce could be more bitter. But to draw
ma per trattar del ben ch'i' vi trovai,	the lesson of good that came my way,
dirò de l'altre cose ch'i' v'ho scorte.	9 I will describe the other things I saw.
Io non so ben ridir com' i' v'intrai,	Just how I entered there I cannot say,
tant' era pien di sonno a quel punto	so full of sleep when I began to veer
che la verace via abbandonai.	12 that I did not see that I had gone astray
	from the one true path.

Dante is lost.

There is no direction to follow in a space that he does not recognize, a place he did not choose to enter. It anguishes him to recall how dire the circumstances were, how confused and terrified he was, so ominous the fear that invades him that death would hardly feel worse. Yet, as he already anticipates (v. 8–9 *ma per trattar del ben ch'i' vi trovai,/dirò de l'altre cose ch'i' v'ho scorte*), Dante will free himself from the condition of bewilderment, developing an awareness and acceptance of his human condition, a condition that is indistinguishably and simultaneously good and bad. It is as mortal as spiritual. It is in the midst of essence and existence, creating a path that is as fallacious as straight. It takes a journey to transform a raw terrifying harsh forest (*oscura selvaggia e aspra*) into an ancient forest (*selva antica*) of lush and of luxuriant foliage (*spessa e viva*).[3] From solitude and isolation into a human experience shared with others. It is a journey of becoming.

We are at the onset of a journey of a human being through life. A human being lost, displaced and terrified of finding himself/herself in a life that is hardly recognizable. It is a shared human experience (*nostra vita*/our lives) as well as this specific person's experience (*mi ritrovai*/I found myself). This is the journey that shakes our understanding, our perception, our way of being with ourselves and with others in this world. It emerges from the collapse of an individual's world as Heidegger[4] discusses in *Being*

---

[3] *Purgatorio*, Canto XXIII, v. 2 and 23.

[4] For an illuminating discussion on the interpretation of Heidegger's concept of world-collapse (being-toward-death) as a collapse of individualized being-in-the-world or the collapse of a culture, see Dreyfus (Dreyfus, 2005). In the context of advanced heart failure experiences, it is important to consider that while we are referring to a collapse of an individual's world, an individual's way of life, his/her family's world also collapses.

and Time (1927/1962): "it is the possibility of the impossibility of every way of comporting oneself toward anything, of every way of existing" (p. 262/307).[5] Anything that had importance, meaning, necessity, place, has lost these connotations. It is a journey requiring transformations of the collapsed world unrecognizable to us (*selva oscura*) into a world that we recognize to be familiar to us (*selva antica*) because anything to which we relate to has importance, meaning, necessity, place; because in it we make sense of who we are.

This is the journey that those who get very sick unwillingly undertake. This is a journey of oneself as a mortal being, hoping for life in the face of death, illness and disease of the self and of the Other (Charmaz, 1995; Moose, 2005).

Mr. Montale, husband, CEO of an international company, 63 years old at the time of heart transplantation. A year earlier, he had undergone aortic valve replacement, but complications required an emergency surgery within 24 hours to implant a Heartmate I Left Ventricular Assist Device (LVAD) to support his badly deteriorated heart pump function until a donor heart becomes available for heart transplantation. Mr. Montale has been on the heart transplantation waiting list for almost 13 months:

> "I was on a business trip and I realized,
> I realized I wasn't walking far.
> I was breathing heavily.
> I was . . . sweating.
> Few days later,
> I could not even keep up with everybody else walking.
> I got scared.
> When I came back my doctor told me to go for a stress test.
> It did not go so well.
> The doctor wanted me to go to a hospital immediately.
> I thought it would be like,
> like my mother. At 80 she had an [aortic] valve surgery
> and in two days she was out of the hospital and fine.
> I?
> I did not get out.
> I don't remember much of that time,

---

[5] We give two sets of page numbers after quoting Heidegger's *Being and Time*; the first refers to pages of the original German version (1927); the second refers to pages in the English translation by Macquarrie and Robinson (1962). We do so because *Being and Time* has been notoriously difficult to translate, as there are also a lot of words created by Heidegger. We have read his work in our respective languages of German and Italian and consulted the English translation of Macquarrie and Robinson to which we refer to here.

about two weeks,
just this:
I was there in the space where they did not know if they were going to save
  me.
Then I got the LVAD."

How to understand Mr. Montale's experiences?

In his longitudinal study of rheumatoid arthritis as chronic illness, Mike Bury, through the narratives of patients' experience shows that the disruption of structures of everyday life, of family relations and of forms of understanding of one's own body, are biographical disruptions (Bury, 1982).

These biographical disruptions have been studied by Kathy Charmaz (1995) as they emerge in different chronic illness conditions. She interprets the experiences of those who suffer from various chronic illnesses including heart and circulatory disease, emphysema, diabetes, multiple sclerosis, chronic fatigue syndrome, and rheumatoid arthritis. Charmaz describes living *with* a chronic disease as developing in stages: one starts experiencing the restrictions imposed by the chronic illness, then one starts making body assessments to identify the trade-offs for revising life goals, commitments and responsibilities in response to the illness constraints and, finally, one surrenders to the sick self, not struggling *against* the illness but *with* the illness.

These, as other studies in sociology of medicine on the experiences of chronic illness point out (e.g., Pierret, 2003), show that what a person can or cannot do in living with a chronic illness becomes familiar in a process of re-elaboration of one's identity.

Let's say that we are walking to a meeting, as Mr. Montale was. While walking, we do not really pay so much attention to the sidewalk leveling, its curves, small holes, our shoes, or for that matter we do not pay attention to our feet, our legs etc., we just walk to go to a meeting, possibly absorbed in a conversation with a colleague, as Mr. Montale was, or thinking about what will happen in the meeting and what we want to get out of it. But what happens if my left foot is in acute pain? Immediately, the foot comes to my attention. It comes to my attention in its function of allowing me to walk and go where I want to go, at the speed most congenial to me. In Heidegger's words, dealing with things we use in the world (tools, equipment etc.), is to relate to something as *Zuhandenheit* (*ready-to-hand*), we just use it without thinking about it while using it, as I do not concentrate on the shoe I wear to walk to a meeting or on the slight curving of the sidewalk. I do not concentrate on my left foot, either. I just walk. Walking the street I take to work, is *familiar*, I just do it — as Heidegger speaks of "that familiarity in accordance with which Dasein [being] as being-with-one-another, 'knows its way about' [*sich auskennt*]" in its public environment (Dreyfus, 1991, p. 103). When the tool malfunctions, is broken or is missing, then we relate to it as *Unzuhandenheit* (*unready-to-hand*). This means that the tool becomes prominent in its function, as a broken shoe would; but also that my left foot in pain becomes prominent as a malfunctioning tool for walking. My foot becomes *auffallend, conspicuous,* in its malfunctioning. Now, I cannot just take a walk in the world going to work oblivious to my shoe, my foot; I feel every step I take. For each step, I can now feel how long the step is, how much I push on my hurting foot and how much the pressure is released when I am standing on the other foot. The other foot is also becoming prominent in my perception of its function of supporting my step. One step opens a new world for me. Things that were transparent to my attention, as my feet were while I was walking to a meeting without pain, are now prominent, *conspicuous* to me. My foot is no longer in the background, *transparent* to my perception of walking to go to a meeting. In its function of allowing me to walk, now malfunctioning, it is prominent, *conspicuous*. My sense of space starts changing, one yard feels so long as if it were a mile, and to walk a yard feels as if it is taking an eternity. Everything around my path (e.g., the ground) changes as my perception of time and space also changes.

What if we apply these concepts to high-tech modern medicine?

In his experience of acute illness, Mr. Montale suddenly realizing that he can "*not even keep up with everybody else walking*", gets scared. He feels threatened in the specific way of experiencing shortness of breath and unusual fatigue. Mr. Montale experiences not only a breathing problem but, in his walk with others he could not keep up with, he experiences something that is wrong with himself, Mr. Montale. This is neither a temporary experience of pain nor the experience of chronic pain Mr. Montale can cope with and learn how to walk with, not struggling *against* it but learning to live *with* it.

Rather, Mr. Montale experiences a temporary breakdown, experiences which Heidegger calls *aufsässig* (obstinate). Going to the doctor and learning about his malfunctioning heart has now brought to the forefront the function that each body part has in allowing him to live. In thinking that he can, with the doctor's help, fix his problem, Mr. Montale experiences the situation as threatening (*"I got scared"*) but still remains in the realm of familiarity as he recognizes it as an experience that his mother also went through (*"I thought it would be like, like my mother. At 80 she had an [aortic] valve surgery and in two days she was out of the hospital and fine"*).

But then, in the hospital, Mr. Montale is helpless with a sense of being threatened in his own existence. He finds himself in a space that is not his own,*"in the space where they did not know if they were going to save me."* Mr. Montale experiences a complete breakdown of his life as the function of his pumping heart is now lost. Heidegger speaks of a tool with a permanent breakdown as *aufdringlich* (obtrusive) (Dreyfus, 1991). Now the body in its entirety has become *conspicuous* with the breakdown of what was so familiar to him, transparent to his perception. This is consistent with what Laura Carstensen (2006) shows is happening when with biographic changes such as age or biographical disruption in acute illnesses, the sense of time is altered and priorities in life change.

"Then I got the LVAD."

Is there a shortcut in high-tech modern medicine?

After the first heart transplantation, performed on December 3, 1967 in Kapstadt by Dr. Christiaan Barnard, the imagination of mankind was captured in an unimaginable way: science, technology and medicine had reached a stage where any diseased organ could be replaced by another one. Mankind was one step closer to immortality. The 'motor exchange', successfully practiced with our cars, was also possible in human beings. Advanced heart failure patients as Mr. Montale are possible candidates for *replacing* their malfunctioning heart with another person's heart (heart transplantation) or with a mechanical circulatory support device, either a Total Artificial Heart or a left ventricular assist device pump implanted (such as an LVAD) which partially *substitutes* the heart pumping function.

False Hope

Ma poi ch'i' fui al piè d'un colle giunto,	But once I had drawn near
là dove terminava quella valle	the bottom of a hill at the far remove,
che m'avea di paura il cor compunto,	15 of the valley that had pierced my heart in fear,

guardai in alto e vidi le sue spalle	I saw its shoulders mantled from above,
vestite già de' raggi del pianeta	by the warm rays of the planet that gives light
che mena dritto altrui per ogne calle. 18	to guide our steps, wherever we may rove.
Allor fu la paura un poco queta,	At last I felt some calming of the fright
che nel lago del cor m'era durata	that had allowed the lake of my heart no rest
la notte ch'i' passai con tanta pieta. 21	while I endured the long and piteous night.
E come quei che con lena affannata,	And as a drowning man with heaving chest
uscito fuor del pelago a la riva,	escapes the current and, once safe on shore,
si volge a l'acqua perigliosa e guata, 24	to see the dangers he has passed,
così l'animo mio, ch'ancor fuggiva,	so did my mind, still lost in flight, once more
si volse a retro a rimirar lo passo	turn back to see the passage that had never
che non lasciò già mai persona viva. 27	let anyone escape alive before.

Dawn has come. Dante looks up toward the sun believing that its natural light will finally unveil to him the path to escape this terrifying affair, removing the blinders of fear and despair. Hope.

If this poem were to be classified as platonic narrative, the model to which narratives in the 14th century were held against, Dante's journey would reach its end in the moment the pilgrim sees the light (Mazzotta, 1979). The experience in Plato's myth (strictly speaking, an analogy) of the cave is grounded in the idea that intellectual contemplation, rational knowledge, and, at the time Dante was writing, knowledge specifically acquired through the study of philosophy, can heal the wounds of the mind and save the otherwise sightless human from the dark abyss of the cave. A Platonic philosopher, knowing how to locate the source of real light, is the only one able to escape the darkness. Others, lured by the flickering light projected on the walls of the cave, would mistake shadows for reality. Knowledge can guide the sightless out of the darkness into the light (Mazzotta, 1993).

Knowledge can take us out of the cave ... does it not sound uncannily familiar to a modern ear?

In contemporary western culture, acquiring scientific knowledge and practicing science with its rational understanding and treatment attends to the intellectual contemplation of issues. The natural sciences and mathematics are able to produce tangible results in the applied sciences, and are sustained by the undeniable scientific and technological advancement following the scientific revolution of the 17th century (Shapin, 1996). Classical science, supported by the continually emerging technology and the production of tangible results in applied sciences, is what saves a human being from dying. It is the 'wagon to eternity' and as such, a sick person needs to surrender to it. The patient must comply.

If I am suddenly very sick, my body is not responding to me as I know it, as I know myself. I am frightened. As in the words of Mr. Montale: *"I could not even keep up with everybody else walking. I got scared."* (v. 5–7 *esta selva selvaggia e aspra e forte/che nel pensier rinova la pàura!/Tant' è amara che poco è più morte;*) I am in the dark and savage wood. My life, as it was, is nowhere in sight, I am powerless. I am lost. Mr. Montale: *"I was there in the space where they did not know if they were going to save me. . . . Can I possibly ever come out of this?"*

In such a situation would I not hope that modern medicine can find the solution to my angst? Would I not rely on the most modern technology and on the medical gaze[6] of the modern knowledgeable doctor to rescue me out of the darkness of such a fearful affair? Of course! Controlled experiments, reproducibility of results, the capacity to resolve complex systems to be investigated into isolable causal chains or units (Engel, 1977) and, yes, the best-kept secret: the hidden assumption of reversibility of time. Ah! Good reliable classical science will return me to my usual life. Yes! Of course, yes! Give me a valve!

Can modern medicine do it?

When a person falls sick and seeks help from a healthcare professional, an encounter within the healthcare system is initiated; the person becomes a patient.

Imagine Dante guided by such wisdom after turning toward the flickering light and discovering that its source is a laboratory light: 'Uhmm, they are testing my blood. They will know all about me, right down to my genes! I can wait here. I can wait for them to tell me who I am!'

No need to write another canto of the Divine Comedy. There is no messy path of becoming, deference to knowledge is required.

Mr. Montale:

> "Then I got the LVAD.
> But when I woke up from LVAD surgery
> oh gosh! I was so weak.

---

[6]Michel Foucault (1994) termed "medical gaze" in the dichotomous body vs. mind paradigm as the dehumanizing understanding of the practice of medicine as a study of the body's pathology separating it from the patient as a person.

I was so weak!
I couldn't walk; it took me a *week* to learn how to sit in *a chair!*
At times you think:
Gee can *I possibly* ever come out of this?
But the staff, the doctor I met and my wife's strength . . .
I came out,
I came out of there."

Mr. Phillips, husband, father, subway conductor, fell ill at the age of 40 with nonischemic dilated cardiomyopathy — a form of muscle disease with reduced heart pump function and enlargement of the heart. Mr. Phillips required the implantation of a mechanical assist device, a Heartmate I LVAD, as a bridge to transplantation and — six weeks later, he underwent successful heart transplantation. Twelve years later, he is hospitalized as the functions of both the transplanted heart and his kidneys are rapidly deteriorating. He remains in the hospital for a full year while waiting for a second heart and simultaneous kidney transplantation:

> "The doctor came in my room and . . .
> and he offered a pump — the LVAD.
> He said 'in your condition it is what you need now'.
> I said no.
> I didn't want this *thing*.
> I was scared.
> I was scared of the unknown.
> I did not know what it was like.
> But I woke up with it.
> I got so sick they implanted it."

Ms. Grahn, mother, sister, realtor, suffered a massive heart attack at age 52 years when a blood-thinning medication was discontinued following coronary artery stent implantation. Although she was immediately placed on a short-term Bi Ventricular Assist Device (BiVAD) and — after transfer to a major transplantation center — on a Heartmate I LVAD, she suffered multi-organ dysfunction syndrome. After recovery, she underwent successful heart transplantation four months later:

> "My heart died.
> I don't remember much.
> I woke up and I had a pump.
> I was scared of it.
> I thought: I'm gonna die with *this*.
> It would go off,
> an alarm,
> and oh! My God!
> What is it?
> Oh my God!
> . . . And it was the battery!

> I had to change the battery!
> I had to learn to *walk*,
> to move.
> I had to learn *my life*."

Mr. Carroll, husband, father, brother, salesman and deer hunter, suffered a catastrophic heart attack at the age of 37, followed by cardiac arrest within weeks. At age 41, he was placed on the USA national waiting list for heart transplantation — the United Network for Organ Sharing (UNOS) waiting list in the Status II urgency category. Being on UNOS II meant Mr. Carroll was able to wait for heart transplantation at home with follow-up visits every one to three months unless worsening symptoms appeared. At the age of 50 years, Mr. Carroll's symptoms worsened and he required a Duraheart LVAD as a bridge to transplantation; four months later he underwent heart transplantation:

> "I was offered an LVAD with Dr. Ozuka
> and I was very *very* apprehensive
> upon meeting Dr. Ozuka [heart surgeon].
> He walked *right* into the room.
> Dr. Ozuka said 'We can do this next Tuesday'.
> Didn't even give me a chance to think about it
> and I was just literally shaken in my boots . . .
> I was like *wow!*
> I do not know if I want this pump.
> I had a vision of a heart,
> a healthy young heart.
> I didn't wanna take the pump.
> They gave me another due date and
> they said this is the day we wanna do it.
> It happened to be my daughter's birthday —
> my seven-year-old.
> I again turned it down and just figured
> if I just leave it alone they will not call me back . . . "

I don't want the pump!

Imagine Dante relying on the power of the knowledgeable rational mind that promises to find the exit of the cave, the promised land, the right choice, the best option; imagine Dante unable to escape the darkness of the cave because he finds himself in a place where there is no direct correspondence between things and their appearance, between things and their meaning. He is lost in the land of dissimilitude — *selva oscura* (Freccero & Jacoff, 1986).

Why lost? These patients did survive the substitution of a valve, the replacement of the heart (Silverstein, 2007). As your *res extensa* has been taken care of by the cardiologist and cardiac surgeon, maybe you would like to talk to a social worker; or maybe to a psychologist to take care of the *res cogitans* and help you deal with your new pump?

If we stand with René Descartes (1986), we know that in order to understand an object, i.e., what it does and what its qualities are, we need to isolate it from its surroundings to study what it purely is. This method of study extends to the study of the subject, to the study of how we understand ourselves. To do this, Descartes states that the self must be isolated from any impression or sense received from the body. If we follow these directives, we can distill the self from the body experience. We can now talk about the journey of illness disjointed from the disease and continue, against Michael Bury's warning (1982), with a separation of cause and meaning where medical thought is identified with disease and lay experience is equated with illness.

And Dante remains lost, and terrified at finding himself in a life that he does not recognize. The hope of being saved is briskly disappointed. When trying to escape the terrifying dark forest, three very real ominous beasts appear on his route to the illuminated hill.

The Body, Being in the World

One of the three beasts, a ravenous she-wolf, keeps pushing Dante back towards the dark wood. The sense of doom, of lost hope, is given both by the movement of Dante's body pushed back step by step and by the translation of light into sound . . . "where the sun is mute" (Cambon, 1970):

tal mi fece la bestia sanza pace,	60 so did I feel as the she-wolf pressed me round,
che, venendomi 'ncontro, a poco a poco	so relentlessly that bit by bit I stepped
mi ripigneval là dove 'l sol tace.	back where the sun is mute on the low ground.

Dante engages the physical senses and their powerful interconnectedness as constitutive of a human experience. The human experiences of fear, of feeling lost, of bewilderment, of temporary relief, or of doom, are elicited in us through physical manifestations. For example, a sense of relief is created through the visual experience of the appearance of a light after a long night in a dark forest or as a calming of the heart rate after having escaped powerful currents: "a drowning man with heaving chest" (v. 22). By the recruitment of the physicality of body experiences as constitutive of the human experience, Dante points to the destitution and insolvency of an isolated rational mind organized to make right choices; a mind unable by itself to define its whereabouts, unable to comprehend the reality around it (Mazzotta, 1979, 1993) (thereby making this reality unfamiliar) and to continue the journey of the person in the here and now.

In encountering Mrs. More in the introduction, we describe some relational experiences of the body in advanced heart failure medical practice: for example the visual experience of nodding, the rhythm of Mrs. More's nods taken as a cue to which the physician responds; the auditory experience, the length of the sound of silences and the repetition of talk setting up a rhythm to follow and to fall into in order to be able to accept death as part of life.[7] Everyone in the room is involved, yes, including the doctor, because it is in participating in the experience with the Other that the doctor makes sense of when to talk, what to repeat, what to add and when to let the silence be; there is no script to follow, no formula for what to say when the doctor responds to Mrs. More's nods, Mrs. More's questions, Mrs. More's gaze.

Making sense of one's own biographical disruptions, as Ms. Grahn, Mr. Montale, Mr. Phillips, and Mr. Carroll recount, starts from bodily experiences of sweating, breathing heavily, not being able to keep up with others walking, or learning to sit, the forceful entrance of a doctor walking "right into the room", of being resuscitated — "my heart died when I woke up

---

[7]Heidegger's notion of communication is relevant here as communication is not only constituted by content, predicates, but by disclosing the salience of what we encounter. "It is letting someone see with us what we have pointed out by way of giving it a definite character. Letting someone see with us shares with the Other that entity which has been pointed out in its definite character. That which is 'shared' is our *being towards* what has been pointed out — a being which we see in common" (Heidegger, 1927/1962, p. 197/155). The communication between Mrs. More and Dr. D of impending death, it is not in the content alone of what Dr. D says but it is a way of accepting, encountering death that needs relational experiences of the body (the visual experience of nodding, the rhythm of Mrs. More's nods as a cue for the physician's response; the auditory experience, the length of the sound of silences and the repetition of talk setting up a rhythm). "Both talking and hearing are based on understanding. And understanding arises neither through talking at length [*vieles Reden*] nor busily hearing something 'all around'. Only he who already understands can listen [*zuhoeren*]. Keeping silent is another essential possibility of discourse, it has the same existential foundation. [...] In talking to one another the person who keeps silent can 'make one understand' [....] Keeping silent is possible only in genuine discoursing. To be able to be silent, *Dasein* must have something to say — that is, must have at his disposal an authentic and rich disclosedness of itself" (Heidegger, 1927/1962, pp. 164–165/208).

with this thing", the pump keeping the body alive: "click clack, click clack", its sound.

These experiences of the body in medical practice are not generalizable under the unspecified umbrellas of illness experience, regardless of whether they are chronic or acute illnesses. Each experience with a specific disease has its own unique manifestations, symptoms, treatments, procedures. As Annemarie Mol (2008) describes in her study of patients with diabetes, pricking one's finger for blood not only constitutes an invasive procedure, but changes the experience of everyday structure. Pricking one's finger is something that patients do to take care of themselves and at the same time it articulates their daily routines. In its specificity, this activity is constitutive of the way in which patients partake in their own care (Mol, 2008). This activity as a monitoring procedure cannot have the same meaning for a patient with advanced heart failure required to undergo biopsy of the heart after heart transplantation to monitor for rejection, as on the biopsy table, partaking in one's own care is not part of the experience (see Chapter 5). The activities one iteratively engages in, as in the case of monitoring the disease, articulates *being* a patient with advanced heart failure or diabetes. As Timmermans and Haas (2008) argue on the necessity to move toward a sociology of disease, in medical practice, patients and clinicians do not lump together the experiences of patients with advanced heart failure, diabetes, HIV, or hypertension. This is because a person who perceives the experience of the disease, of its physiological constraints and of its treatment, is living *this* specific experience. This is also a body that is claimed as one's own, as Mr. Montale, Ms. Grahn, Mr. Phillips, Mr. Carroll, and Mrs. More each recognizes theirs as being Mr. Montale, Ms. Grahn, Mr. Phillips, Mr. Carroll, and Mrs. More, the body, being in the world. Accepting this is a first step of moving beyond the forms of dualism (disease vs. illness; mind vs. body) with which illness narratives and models of best practices (Charon, 2001; Stewart *et al.*, 2003; Tresolini & Pew-Fetzer Task Force, 1994) had to contend to overcome the reduction to a biomedical level (disease) and creating other ways of knowing, further dissecting the person's experience.

We consider in this book the experiences in advanced heart failure practice, anchored in the body with its specific physiological constraints, with the manifestations of the disease and with demands of integration of scientific and technological advances of high-tech modern medicine into persons' lives.

Mr. Phillips: *"he offered a pump — the LVAD. . . . I didn't want this thing. . . . I was scared of the unknown. I did not know what it was like."*

LVAD, BiVAD, disease, the body: Conspicuousness and obtrusiveness in high-tech modern medicine

Although changes in modern treatment options over the last 15 years are prolonging the lives of advanced heart failure patients (Cubbon *et al.*, 2011), more than in other chronic diseases, the prognosis for these patients remains uncertain, not so on statistical grounds but at the level of the individual person as shown in Figure 1.1 by the progression trajectories of different diseases. Making the course of this life-threatening disease unpredictable (Allen *et al.*, 2012 and reference therein) is its dramatically and not linearly fluctuating clinical course across the spectrum of the disease (Lanken *et al.*, 2008 and as also shown in Figure 1.1). This includes the possibility of unexpected sudden death due to chaotic fibrillation of the ventricles also called lethal arrhythmia. Patients in advanced heart failure for whom

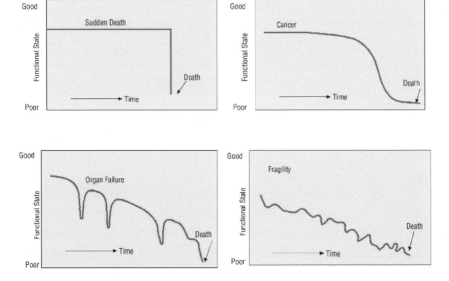

Figure 1.1: Disease progression trajectories in sudden death, cancer, organ failure (for example heart failure), and fragility (= frailty). Note the various modes of disease progression, specifically the uncertainty of prognosis associated with organ failure (left lower figure) (modified after Martínez-Sellés *et al.*, 2009).

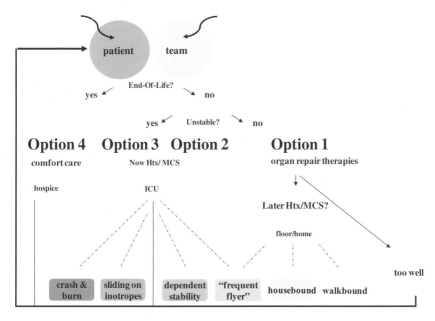

Figure 1.2: Recurring heart failure patient/team encounter and decision-making about treatment options 1–4. Note the increasing severity of the heart failure syndrome as indicated by the boxes on the botton of the figure from right to left, indicating "too well, walkbound, housebound, frequent flyer (frequent hospital re-admission), dependent stability (stable on inotropic medication), sliding on inotropes, crash & burn"; Htx (Heart Transplant); MCS (Mechanical Circulatory Support) (adapted from Deng and Naka, 2007, details see text).

remission into less symptomatic disease is unlikely (Hunt *et al.*, 2009) face four different treatment options possibly unfolding (Figure 1.2). All four options have a significant impact on the patient's and family's daily lives. The first three have the combined goal of improving the patients' survival as well as their quality of life. The fourth option focuses on quality of life exclusively. Due to the complexity of the clinical course (Figure 1.1) of advanced heart failure, these options are not always mutually exclusive, that is, for example, Option 2, as described below, can be a treatment option after Option 3.

Option 1: Cardiac repair strategies: optimal medical management with comprehensive lifestyle changes, including (a) swallowing of neurohormonal antagonist medicines such as beta-adrenergic receptor blockers and renin-angiotensin-aldosterone antagonists to block the adverse effects of stress hormones and kidney hormones that are chronically activated in advanced heart failure (Adigopula *et al.*, 2014). These medications have side effects ranging from dizziness to worsening of the patients' kidney function; (b) cardiac resynchronization therapy (implantation of specialized pace-makers) with the function of synchronizing the heart's electrical activity; (c) reparative therapies delivered via a cardiac catheter including coronary artery stent implantation or valve implantation and cardiac surgery including coronary artery bypass grafting and valve repair or replacement; and (d) implantation of a cardioverter-defibrillator, an internal pulse generator encased in a small titanium cover that senses electrical activity in the myocardium. When pathological cardiac arrhythmia is sensed, the cardioverter-defibrillator delivers strong, potentially life-saving, internal instantaneous electrical shocks to the myocardium. Felt by the patient, these shocks may produce fear and anxiety, insomnia, feelings of loss of control and thus affect relationships and sexual activities (Palacios Ceña *et al.*, 2011) and reference therein).

Option 2: Cardiac support strategies: Open heart surgery with implantation of mechanical circulatory support devices: (a) the Left or Right Ventricular Assist Device, (LVAD or RVAD) or Biventricular Assist Device (BiVAD), mechanical pumps that help pump blood from the main chambers of the heart (the left and right ventricles) to the rest of the body (Deng & Naka, 2007). The mechanical circulatory support device inserted in the patient's body is connected through a driveline out of the patient's belly wall, to an external portable set composed of two rechargeable batteries and a small computer. A second strategy is the implantation of the Total Artificial Heart. This mechanical device, made of polyurethane, substitutes for the patient's heart, which in turn is removed and disposed of. The weight of these systems varies from 3 pounds (1–1.5 kilograms), in the case of a biventricular assist device (BiVAD) (Figure 1.3) or LVAD (Figure 1.4), to 13 pounds (5–6 kilograms) in the case of the Total Artificial Heart system (Figure 1.5).

A mechanical circulatory support device is offered as a 'bridge to heart transplantation' (Option 3) when a patient is at very high risk of dying while waiting for a heart offer, as in the cases of worsening of cardiac pump function, of secondary organ dysfunction or of development of lethal arrhythmias. Being a major surgery, implantation of any of these devices requires that a patient who undergoes such procedure be temporarily removed from the active heart waiting list until having completely recovered

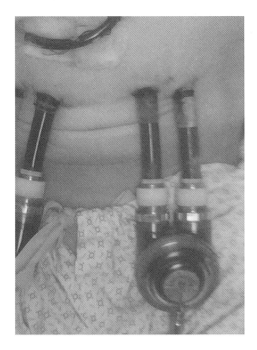

Figure 1.3: Mr. James with his BiVAD closeup. Note both inflow- and outflow cannulas of the RVAD and LVAD exiting the abdominal wall to be connected with power supply and computer (details see text, Chapter 2).

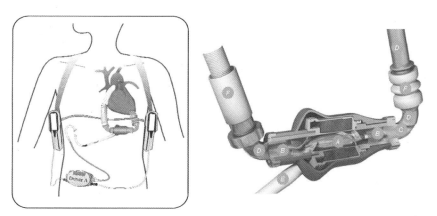

Figure 1.4: Heartmate II Left Ventricular Assist Device (Thoratec Inc, Pleasanton, CA): The rotary pump is placed inside the body near the heart, receiving blood from the left ventricle and propelling it into the aorta. The patient's heart can continue to contribute to the overall heart and circulation activity. The rotary pump is connected through the driveline, sticking out the belly wall, with a small computer (controller) and two batteries positioned in belts across the patient's shoulders (details see text).

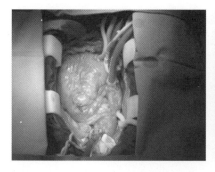 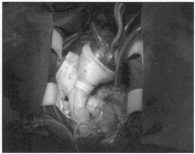

Figure 1.5: Total Artificial Heart (Syncardia Systems Inc, AZ), viewed from the patient's head in the operating room: The Total Artificial Heart replaces the patient's own heart (left) and takes over left and right heart function (right) (details see text).

(UNOS Status 7: "Temporarily not transplantable"). This often provokes considerable anxiety in patients and their families for fear of not being fully recovered when the 'right' heart becomes available (see Option 3).

As in the case of patients agreeing to have an implantable cardioverter-defibrillator (Matlock, Nowels, & Bekelman, 2010, p. 824) and as Ms. Grahn, Mr. Montale, Mr. Phillips and Mr. Carroll experienced, having a mechanical circulatory support device implanted in their body, is always very difficult because of the prospect of a life with a machine, a titanium pump, in the body pumping the heart: *"I felt like I was a science experiment, and it sparked a bit of fear in me to say the least!"* (Deng & Naka, 2007, p. 348).

Anxiety and fear is also experienced by the family members as a decision must often be made unexpectedly and rapidly because a loved one had just coded:[8] *"I watched the nurse assigned to him [husband] after surgery operate this console and about 27 different bags and bottles going into his neck, groin, chest — every orifice. And I thought: What have I done? He's on a respirator, so I can't ask him!"* (*Ibid.*, p. 374). The recovery from mechanical circulatory support device implantation surgery can be slow, often very painful and with contrasting if not conflicting feeling about the

---

[8] 'Coded' is a medical term used to indicate a high status emergency of a hospitalized patient dying and most often in need of resuscitation. We use it here because many patients in advanced heart failure quickly learn to use it, having experienced it more than once. It is important to note that patients would refer to "having died" as analogous to the term 'coded'.

life with a machine. It is welcomed after being very sick for a long time: *"For the first time in months, I could walk for extended periods without being out of breath. I could eventually taste my food and generally felt better than I had in at least 3 years. However, the recovery period from the surgery was quite painful. The LVAD was to remain implanted until such time as I could receive a heart transplant, for which I had previously qualified and was at Level 1B" (Ibid., p. 373).* It is also very complex for patient and their family who have to learn a completely new life, entirely dependent on the good functioning of the mechanical circulatory support:

"My wife was very troubled by the device and the possibility that we would lose the electrical power necessary to run the pump." "A car wreck just up the road from us had taken out a power line." And as Mr. James reports: *"This tube sticking out my belly here connects to this set with a computer and, and two batteries ... eh the batteries! They have to be recharged every 2 to 4 hours. You mustn't forget, or well, ... you are not ... no more. At night, when I go to sleep I am plugged into an electric wall outlet like a TV set."*

As we saw at the beginning of the chapter, patients, with the help of family caregivers, must learn how to wash their body, how to avoid wetting the computer or causing infection where the driveline from the computer enters their body; no swimming, no boat riding, and many other things they used to do. New ones to come: *"The LVAD is not conducive to the most romantic of sex lives. As the pace mounts, so does the noise. The first time, I was convinced that he would expire before he ever reached a climax. After a while, we became less anxious. What with drivelines, power lines, and batteries, the whole act could resemble a comedy routine" (Ibid., p. 328).* Altered sexual relationships do create feelings of guilt in the ill person: *"My wife and I attempted to have sex. I wore the battery packs to give me more flexibility, but that proved to be dangerous as I bruised my wife with them. So, I quickly unplugged them and connected myself to the charger. Now, I was limited to a 5-foot radius from the equipment" (Ibid., p. 334).*

The "click clack, click clack, click clack" mechanical sound of the assist device maintaining the rhythm of a human's heartbeat also has emotionally disturbing effects on others: *" ... to lay people [the LVAD] is kind of freakish. People who see Carl now comment on how disturbed they were by the noise the pump made (his hairstylist, tailor, dentist, dermatologist, etc.) ... "*

(*Ibid*, p. 375). However, explaining to others how a BiVAD works, how it is implanted, how it is functioning, can contribute to a self-elaboration of both the physical and the emotional experience of life with machines as evolving biography.

Option 3: Cardiac replacement strategies: heart transplantation (the Total Artificial Heart described under Option 2 is a heart replacement also, however in advanced heart failure practice it is discussed always in the context of mechanical assist devices). The donor heart completely replaces the patient's heart, which in turn is removed and disposed of. As with Option 2, this option also requires open heart surgery. It has a survival rate of 85%–90% during the first year after transplant. Living with the donor heart requires taking high doses of immunosuppressant medicines because the body recognizes somebody else's heart as a foreign body and attacks it. It is a very complex and fine balance between minimizing the risk of rejection and minimizing the morbidity associated with the adverse effects of immunosuppressive drugs: a high likelihood of infections, which the immune system, so depressed, cannot fight and an increased long-term probability of developing cancer. The standard procedure used for rejection surveillance is the endomyocardial biopsy. This invasive, painful, expensive procedure which has a 0.5%–1.5% case morbidity (Deng *et al.*, 2006) involves accessing the patient's heart through the jugular vein in order to remove and analyze a small sample of heart tissue. This procedure is repeated frequently after heart transplantation, as described in Chapter 5. While maintaining a rigorous schedule of visits with their physician, heart transplant patients must also learn to monitor their own bodies for any sign of potential rejection and infection, both potentially fatal.

While making sense of new symptoms indicating possible rejection, infection or organ dysfunction, patients often embrace the new heart as a gift (Healy, 2006) and as if it had a personality. They talk about the heart as if it had a soul, a history, a biography that would allow it to understand that it has a 'new home'. It is the heart after all, since the Middle Ages, that has occupied a place in people's imagination, in poetry, songs and everyday talk, as a secret place where love is produced, the place where the soul originates and performs its operation (Webb, 2010).

Option 4: Cardiac repair strategies with the predominant goal of improving quality of life: less aggressive, quality-of-life emphasizing palliative therapy is an option more common in the case of elderly patients, but it is also a very real possibility for younger patients with advanced heart failure for whom life-prolonging options such as heart transplantation or destination (lifetime) mechanical circulatory support are not possible. Even more prominent than in the cases of the other options, the discourse and practice in which patients and their families participate in high-tech modern medicine is rooted in a 'death-denying' society (Zimmermann, 2007). Faced with their own personal struggles of making sense of and accepting death as part of life, advanced heart failure patients face additional complex physical and emotional struggles. Planning for palliative care can create conflicts when the therapeutic option desired by the patient is not aligned with the family's preferred one or with medical possibilities/realities proposed by the physician (Allen *et al.*, 2012). This situation can shake up family structure and relations which in turn affects the kind of the individual experience at the end of life (Broom & Kirby, 2013). A medical philosophy and culture focusing almost exclusively on curing illness and prolonging life (Morrison & Meier, 2004), has prevented an equal improvement of care that supports quality of life and relief of suffering (Chattoo & Atkin, 2009; Gott *et al.*, 2008; O'Leary *et al.*, 2009), and provides support for all stakeholders in accepting death as part of life. Caught in this dichotomized context (Morrison & Meier, 2004), patients rarely have conversations about death with their physician (Low *et al.*, 2011). This is particularly grave because as their illness progresses and patients' experiences with the disease change, preferences, too, may change. Krumholz *et al.* (1998) reported a study where 178 of 936 patients with advanced heart failure had changed their preferences for resuscitation within two months. In a later study, Krumholz and coworkers (Goldstein *et al.*, 2004) report that not having conversations about quality of life and death between patients with implanted cardioverter defibrillators (Option 1) and physicians resulted in patients receiving shocks from the implanted cardioverter defibrillators during the last month of life or even a few minutes before death.

Embodied human experiences: Loss of significance in high-tech modern medicine

The embodied human experiences of an individual in the interactions with technological advancements of modern medicine make the entire experience specific, as the course of the advanced heart failure disease is unpredictable and fluctuating non-linearly across the spectrum of possibilities (Figures 1.1 and 1.2). Patients and their families' lives are disrupted and *familiarity* with what was known has broken down (Heidegger, 1927/1962). As one's body or loved one's body becomes so *conspicuous* in its malfunctioning, the functional aspect of the body becomes more evident. In the moments of fear for one's own life, or fear of losing the loved one, the *conspicuousness* of a malfunctioning body, now so evident in its function to sustain life, discloses the body as an instrument that has failed to do its job. The body now is malfunctioning with permanently broken down (obtrusive, *aufdringlich*) part(s). This gaze on the broken down body parts, not as a whole 'me', is part of the experience of patients and their families facing one of those options. When these options are discussed as biomedical options, a gaze into the properties of the heart and body, as well as their natural functions is possible; it is a gaze into what biomedical sciences study (i.e., the heart's properties and its function/malfunctions in the biological life of a human being). This is a gaze into what Heidegger calls *present-at-hand* (i.e., something's property and its natural functions). It is something that has been stripped of its role, its meaning in the person's relation in the world, the *ready-to-hand*. Patients (as Mr. Carroll, Mr. Phillips and Mr. Montale experienced), do not make decisions based on a gaze on the heart properties or function, but, as doctors often recognize, patients make decisions when they can have a sense of what it could mean in their lives. As Mr. Phillips recounts when he had coded and was implanted with an LVAD: "*I said no. I didn't want this thing. I was scared. I was scared of the unknown. I did not know what it was like. But I woke up with it. I got so sick they implanted it*". This means that patients do not experience the broken part in an intact body, but they experience the entire body broken. In contrast to the examples that Heidegger speaks of in our dealing with equipment and tools, the experience of patients with a failing organ, for example a failing heart, is both of a broken tool and of a threat to one's existence. These are inseparable.

It is in uncovering the functional aspects of one's body — or of the loved one's body — as *unready-to-hand* that it is possible to accept the idea of a substitution of a permanently broken organ (obtrusive) by heart transplantation or a substitution of part of the heart's pumping function by LVAD/BiVAD implantation.

At this point, the issue becomes the following: how does one makes sense of the world, either with a heart from another person substituting one's own heart or attached to a machine that substitutes the person's heart's function; as we said the experience is of threat to one's existence.

Ms. Kirsch: *I watched the nurse assigned to him [husband] after surgery operate this console and about 27 different bags and bottles going into his neck, groin, chest — every orifice. And I thought: What have I done? He's on a respirator, so I can't ask him!*

Ms. Grahn: *I woke up and I had a pump. I was scared of it. I thought: I'm gonna die with this. It would go off, an alarm, and oh! My God! What is it? Oh my God! . . . And it was the battery! I had to change the battery! I had to learn to walk, to move. I had to learn my life.*

Mr. Montale: *Then I got the LVAD. But, when I woke up from LVAD surgery, oh gosh! I was so weak. I was so weak! I couldn't walk; it took me a week to learn how to sit in a chair! At times you think: Gee can I possibly ever come out of this?*

For Ms. Grahn, Mr. Montale, as well as for Ms. Kirsch, there is a breakdown of the relational aspect of one's life — what Heidegger calls *significance* (*Bedeutsamkeit*). In advanced heart failure, as a person uncovers him/herself as made of replaceable body parts, this breakdown extends to the system of relations that gives significance of one's own life as Ms. Grahn says, of one's being-in-the-world. In Mr. Montale's experience, for example, entering in his office, sitting in his chair in the morning, is part of the relations with spaces, activities and things, that he does in order to do his work, in order to be the CEO of an international company. Here, a chair is equipment *ready-to-hand*, the chair is what Mr. Montale uses without thinking about it; he enters his office, maybe the phone is already ringing and, reaching for it, he sits in his chair. At home, sitting in a chair to eat at a family dinner is something Mr. Montale also just does. Here he sits to enjoy, as a person, as a husband, a delicious family dish that his beloved wife has cooked. All these relations held together make up Mr. Montale's world, its significance. A relational web binds physical things, equipment and persons together into a meaningful whole. The chair in which Mr. Montale sits to have dinner with his wife is for Mr. Montale meaningfully webbed in a context-specific way with the table where the plates in which the food is served are placed, with the room next to the kitchen he designed with his wife. Each of these tools and spaces, the chair, the plate, the dining room, the house signifies (*bedeuten*) the other tools' role for Mr. Montale.

"*Then I got the LVAD*". What is the *significance*, the meaningful relational web of an LVAD? It is not meaningfully webbed to anything that is not the hospital, the hospital bed, the doctors and the nurses. With the LVAD there is a breakdown of the relational web that binds physical things, equipment and persons together into a meaningful whole, a breakdown of *significance*. Coping with the LVAD is not an activity embedded in a *familiar* world where Mr. Montale can recognizes himself being a husband, a CEO, a person who likes his wife's home cooking. As for now it is experienced as a breakdown of significance, a breakdown of 'the background upon which entities can have sense and activities can have a point" (Dreyfus, 1991, p. 97).

And now, to sit in a chair is different, "*it took me a week to learn how to sit in a chair*". It does not have those relations to other things, to people, to known life any longer and Mr. Montale's world now is not *familiar* anymore. After waking up from the implantation surgery, to sit in a chair is no longer using *ready-to-hand* equipment without thinking about it, transparently, but a goal. His body, as he knew it, as he knew his world, is not recognizable as 'me'. The embodied understanding of what counts as real has changed. Living with advanced heart failure and taking care of a patient with advanced heart failure are experiences at the frontier, in the *selva oscura*, in the land of dissimilitude. It is the experience of a world that has collapsed, as it has lost its *significance*, leaving us without possibility of making sense, recalling, recognizing what we had known. There, Martin Heidegger (1927/1962) says that we are alone. Yes, we are. It is true, we cannot understand the land of dissimilitude through the experience of another person living it. We cannot experience and therefore cannot fully make sense of Mr. Montale's experience. We can only capture that the experience can exist for all humans, that is, we understand it as a human experience. Yet, the experiences in the land of dissimilitude, "*I was there in the space where they did not know if they were going to save me*", are not unfolding in an isolated space:

The Encounter

Mentre ch'i' rovinava in basso loco,	And as I drove myself into the depth,
dinanzi a li occhi mi fu offerto	a shape was offered to my vision, wan
chi per silenzio parea fioco.	63 as if from a long silence it had kept.

There, in the land of dissimilitude, Dante receives a gift (*v. 62 mi fu offerto*). The ultimate gift: the capacity to recognize and relate to another being. Dante recognizes him through the shared human experience.

Quando vidi costui nel gran diserto,	Seeing him in that great desert, I began,
"Miserere di me" gridai a lui	to call out. *"Miserere*-on me" I cried,
"qual che tu sii, od ombra od omo certo!"	66 "whatever you are, a shade or a solid man!"
Rispousemi: " non omo, omo già fui,	"Not man; although I was a man," he replied
e li parenti miei furon lomabrdi,	"My parents were both Mantuans. I descend
mantoani per patrïa ambedui.	69 from those of Lombardy on either side.
Nacqui sub Iulio, ancor che fosse tardi,	I was born *sub Julio*, at the latter end.
e vissi a Roma sotto 'l buon Augusto	Under the good Augustus I lived at Rome,
nel tempo de li dei falsi e bugiardi.	72 in the days when false and lying gods still reigned.
Poeta fui e cantai di quell giusto	I was a poet, and I sang of him,
figliuol d'Anchise che venne di Troia,	Anchises's righteous son, who sailed from Troy
poi che 'l superbo Iïón fu combusto.	75 after the burning of proud Ilium.
Ma perché tu ritorni a tanta noia?	But why do you turn back toward trouble?

Dante meets Virgil. He meets Virgil who will be his guide through a good part of his journey. Dante meets Virgil the poet (v. 74), not a proponent of a knowledge with its power of abstraction and its universal laws capable of illuminating the patterns of human life (Mazzotta, 1999). Why not? Well let's try now that we have more of a sense for the forest. When "it is not in our power to discern the truest opinions", Descartes suggests:

> ... imitating travelers who, finding themselves lost in some forest, should not wander about turning this way and that, nor, worse still, stop in one place, but should always walk in as straight a line as they can in one direction and never change it for feeble reasons, even if at the outset it had perhaps been only chance that made them choose it, for by this means, even if they are not going exactly where they wish, at least they will eventually arrive somewhere where they will probably be better off than in the middle of a forest (p. 14).

Yet, in the land of dissimilitude there is no direct correspondence between things and their appearance. What is the straight line from having my heart 'removed and disposed of'? How do I walk in a straight line when living with another person's heart? What does a straight line look like from here?

These questions have absolutely no meaning. They are gibberish, nonsensical talk, to a person in the land of dissimilitude and also for those outside it. They are meaningless because we organize them in a context of a method, specifically a method to get out of the forest. From the mountain (v. 13 *Ma poi ch'i' fui al piè d'un colle giunto*) illuminated by the fugacious light showing the straight path through the mountain of *Purgatorio* to *Paradiso*, Dante, rather than up the mountain, will go down to the Inferno, through the center of the Earth, exiting on the opposite side, on the south pole, and find himself in the forest around the same mountain that was originally impossible to climb. There, rather than in the *selva oscura,* he finds himself in the ancient forest (*selva antica*) with lush and luxuriant foliage (*spessa e viva)* in Purgatorio.[9] Dante does not leave the *selva oscura*, he transforms it. From solitude, fear and isolation of the *selva oscura* into a human experience shared with others of the *selva antica*. There is no formula, no method to look for because the question is not how to get out of the forest but how to make it one's own. Yet, the answer Dante gives is: not alone. There is only shared human experience, resonating humanity that allows one who is lost and the Other to recognize one another. Dante replenishes the disillusioned intellectual promises of Platonic philosophy with those promises offered by poetry: preserving individuality, reinstituting the emotions and the body as integral to the human shared experience. To the despair of the Platonic philosopher, alone in the land of dissimilitude, Dante responds with hope (Mazzotta, 1979), the hope that can come only from a human experience shared with the Other (Buber, 2013; Levinas, 1979).

Virgil introduces himself by telling Dante where and when he was born, where he lived and where his parents were from; he collocates his life in the historical and political context (v. 69–73) and, finally, identifies himself as a poet. Virgil introduces himself as a *person*. Dante meets Virgil, a person with all his irreducible identities and historicity. And there is hope.

Ms. Mereau, mother, wife, sister, daughter, intensive care nurse, at 49 years developed rapid onset heart failure and was diagnosed with giant cell myocarditis likely as a rare autoimmune response to vaccination, cardiac arrested four times and underwent urgent heart transplantation:

> It was completely non-verbal, you [the doctor] were attentive, you listened, you responded to what I said, you didn't discount anything I said, you were not in a hurry, you didn't have another agenda, you were not anxious to leave the room and let me die alone which is what I had the impression the other people . . . just couldn't wait to get out of my presence because then it was kind of like they

---

[9]*Purgatorio*, Canto XXIII, v. 2 and 23.

weren't responsible for me. Then of course when you touched me, I mean no one had touched me, even Jack [her husband] was afraid to touch me, he told me afterwards particularly the night in the emergency room when I felt like I was on fire and I said don't touch me. But that was different, he was afraid he would hurt me. The other doctors, I had the sense were afraid of being involved. You weren't afraid of me dying. You were going to do everything in your power to help me, but you also weren't . . . you weren't in charge of whether I lived or whether I died, God was. I was perfectly comfortable with that, you were perfectly comfortable with that.

This is the encounter of two humans as mortal beings hoping for life in the face of death. They are confronted with illness and disease of the body as one's own reality, as the irreducible historicity of oneself. As anticipated in the initial verses (v. 8–9 *ma per trattar del ben ch'i' vi trovai,/dirò de l'altre cose ch'i' v'ho scorte*), through the encounter with Virgil in Canto I, and, with his help throughout the Inferno to Purgatorio and the garden of Eden, Dante will free himself from the condition of bewilderment and displacement as he develops an awareness and acceptance of his human condition, as familiarity with his life that is indistinguishably both good and bad, both physical and spiritual, where illness and disease are irreducibly integrated as human experience. It is as mortal as spiritual, following a path that is as fallacious as straight. It will take a journey with the Other:

E io a lui: ≪Poeta, io ti richeggio per quello Dio che tu conoscesti, acciò ch'io fugga questo male e peggio,	*130* "Poet," I said to him "so that I may escape this harm and worse that may await, in the name of that God you never knew, I pray
che tu mi meni là dov'or dicesti, sì ch'io veggia la porta di san Pietro e color cui tu fai cotanto mesti≫. Allor si mosse, e io li tenni dietro.	you lead me out to see Saint Peter's gate and all those souls that you have told me of, who must endure their miserable state." I followed him as he began to move.

It will take a journey with the Other to recognize himself (Paradiso v. 131). And Dante's heart, freed from fear is filled with sweetness (Paradiso v. 63). The heart, what an attuned symbolism for this very book's content!

The Status Quo

So what is the status quo? We start from the predicament that if we accept that a person falling sick finds him/herself in the land of dissimilitude as in the experience of a person with advanced heart failure, then s/he will have to learn to live and interpret a life with an artificial heart, with an LVAD, with a BiVAD, with the heart from somebody else. S/he will have to make sense of, recall, relate to things that are not recognizable as they were before. It is neither the self (as a conscious sense of who we are as persons) nor the body (as the organic parts) separately needing to be taken care of. It is a transformation of a collapsed world into one that has significance and therefore is familiar to the persons taking the journey. It is in the actions, in relation with others, with things old and now new, like taking a shower, walking, sitting, eating, talking, listening, where the new, the unknown becomes familiar and owned. This is not a path where one can venture alone. While in the experience of the land of dissimilitude one is alone, one is not isolated. This is our status quo: The practice of high-tech modern medicine becomes the particularly powerful domain in which integration of science, technology, body and personhood takes place; it requires learning for the purpose of guiding integration of treatments, goals and technological advancement into *this specific person's* life.

Yes, nobody said it would be easy.

CHAPTER 2
THE ROOTS FOR *PERSON*CARE

Mr. James had been a healthy, physically active young man until he developed advanced heart failure about ten years ago. Now in his thirties, his condition has deteriorated dramatically. Several days ago, he was emergently hospitalized and resuscitated, after having suffered a fast chaotic heartbeat (lethal arrhythmia). For the past years, Mr. James has been struggling with the idea of receiving a heart transplant. Without intervention, he is facing imminent death, either from decompensated heart failure[1] or from another episode of fast chaotic heartbeat with repeated firing and battery exhaustion of his internal cardioverter-defibrillator (see Option 1 in Chapter 1) for which he has been hospitalized. Mr. James opts for heart transplantation; he is placed in the highest urgency category on the USA national waiting list for heart transplantation — the United Network for Organ Sharing (UNOS) waiting list. However, based on the risk of another potentially fatal lethal arrhythmia, his advanced heart failure healthcare team suggests the implantation of a BiVAD as a bridge to transplantation in the event that another of these serious arrhythmia episodes with loss of consciousness occurs. Mr. James remains hospitalized in intensive care under close monitoring, waiting for a donor heart.

A lethal arrhythmia does occur, much sooner than expected, and the BiVAD is implanted (Figures 1.3 and 2.1) in an emergency surgery. Mr. James recovers from the BiVAD implantation surgery in the Cardiothoracic Intensive Care Unit (CTICU). The clinical course of his recovery is impressive. He is extubated on Day 1 after the operation, and on Day 2 he is able to sit in a chair and starts physical therapy, a major achievement after

---

[1] Heart failure is the state in which the heart is unable to pump sufficient oxygenated blood to match the oxygen requirements of the body. Decompensated heart failure is the state in which the compensatory mechanisms of the body are inadequate to deal with the inability of the heart to pump and the person suffering from it develops symptoms such as retention of water in the lungs and the legs.

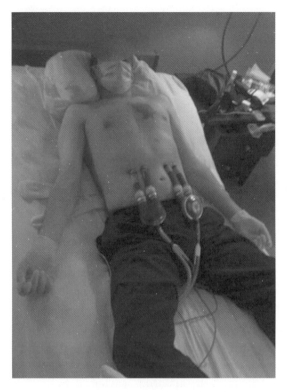

Figure 2.1: Mr. James with his BiVAD at home where his parents are changing the exit site dressings under sterile conditions. Note both inflow- and outflow cannulas of the RVAD and LVAD exiting the abdominal wall to be connected with power supply and computer (details see text).

assist device implantation as other patients report (Chapter 1). The plan is for Mr. James to completely recover from the BiVAD surgery and preferably to be discharged home from the hospital to get into the best possible shape for the transplant surgery.

Dr. D has been the attending physician from the first day of Mr. James' BiVAD implantation (Day 0) and rounds on a daily basis for a consecutive fourteen-day period.

Since Day 5, Mr. James has been experiencing problems in sleeping, since Day 6, pain in his legs and since Day 8, symptoms of fluid overload. These problems are impairing his ability to participate in the physical activities necessary for his recovery: getting out of bed, weighing himself, walking and sitting in a chair to allow for a different distribution of fluid in the lungs to prevent pneumonia. The physical therapy regimen (walking, eating, etc.) is important to increase his body mass, including muscle mass and his physical strength; this is of particular importance for Mr. James because secondary to the progression of his advanced heart failure syndrome he has lost more than 40 pounds (20 kg) and is suffering from a condition called cachexia. Cachexia is the final common pathway of different diseases such advanced heart failure or cancer, mediated by white blood cells through a systemic inflammatory activation initiating catabolic pathways in the body, deconstructing proteins, reducing body mass, producing loss of appetite, and loss of weight; it is associated with a high mortality risk (von Haehling & Anker, 2013). The BiVAD surgery Mr. James has undergone can temporarily induce or worsen this condition. For Mr. James to recover, the condition must reverse.

On Day 10 postoperatively, Dr. D enters:

Day 10

1	Dr. D:	Hi young man.
2	Mr. James:	Hi!
3	Dr. D:	How is life?
4	Mr. James:	Getting better. Had a nice breakfast.
5	Dr. D:	I saw you. *(3 s)*
6	Mr. James:	Got the eggs.
7		Got the turkey sandwich.
8		Got a nice little fruit cup.
9		My feet are starting to feel a little bit better.
10		*(5.5 s)*
11	Dr. D:	That's good news.
12	Mr. James:	Yes it is.
13		I got my fingers crossed,
14		so hopefully I will be going for a walk soon.
15	Dr. D:	Beautiful! *(2.7 s)*

Beautiful! As he did in the situation when he learned about Mr. Rice taking a shower (Chapter 1), Dr. D exclaims (line 15) 'Beautiful!' upon learning about Mr. James eating a fruit cup and his intention to resume walking in the corridor.

Dr. D feels that despite pain and fluid overload Mr. James is making progress. In CoGen sessions, reflecting on the way Mr. James describes his lunch, Dr. D says: "there is something in the way he said it that I could resonate with, in other words, I could almost taste the turkey sandwich and the fruit cup." It is a physical experience, the pleasure in eating that is communicated and forms the basis for Dr. D's impression that Mr. James' cachexia is reversing: "Someone with worsening cachexia does not talk like this about food." In addition to using the word 'nice' twice (lines 4 and 8) to describe the pleasure in eating his meal, Mr. James, in response to Dr. D's question (line 3), chose his breakfast as the first information to share with Dr. D.

Mr. James will report about the pain in his legs and his difficulty in sleeping after the direct inquiry of Dr. D:

15	Dr. D:	Beautiful! *(2.7s)*
16		And did you get some sleep?
17	Mr. James:	Ah I got a little bit of sleep, not much.
18	Dr. D:	Mm hmm.
19	Mr. James:	My legs were just so sore last night.
20		It was just kind of hard to sleep.
21		But they are starting to feel a little bit better right now.
22		*(3s)*
23	Dr. D:	Who is going to walk with you?

So why not ask Mr. James immediately about the pain and the sleepless night, after acknowledging having seen Mr. James eating earlier (line 5), since all these appear to be pressing issues? Dr. D (line 5) does not add anything, does not ask anything. Silence. Three seconds of silence is a long silence considering that most long silence interval durations cluster around the one second interval (0.9–1.2 s) (Jefferson, 1989). After these three seconds of silence, either Dr. D or Mr. James could have continued the conversation without disrupting the flow and the medical encounter. For example, the question Dr. D asks at line 16 could have been asked right after the silence after line 5. Let's see what that would look like:

1	*Dr. D:*	*Hi young man.*
2	*Mr. James:*	*Hi!*
3	*Dr. D:*	*How is life?*
4	*Mr. James:*	*Getting better. Had a nice breakfast.*
5	*Dr. D:*	*I saw you.*
16		And did you get some sleep?
17	Mr. James:	Ah I got a little bit of sleep, not much.

Interestingly, making line 16 follow line 5, thereby omitting the conversation about food from which Dr. D assesses that cachexia is reversing, does not require the silence on line 5 (Schegloff, 2007). This sequence makes sense but stresses problem presentation as commonly seen in primary care practice (Heritage & Maynard, 2006). 'I am the doctor, I need to cure your body. What is the problem?' This is not what is happening in Dr. D's and Mr. James' encounter.

In their encounter, there is a silence on line 5, after which Mr. James continues talking about his meal. Dr. D allows silence, which signals to Mr. James that he is listening and the topic is possibly not concluded. Dr. D, entering Mr. James' room, has two objectives during the encounter. The first objective is to see how Mr. James is feeling and how his recovery is proceeding. The second objective is to make sure that the steps toward recovery are available for Mr. James to take. Let's discuss the two objectives further. First objective: signaling that Dr. D is listening can, as it does, move Mr. James to continue to talk. This is already an important prompt, because Mr. James, who is usually very communicative as in this encounter, has not always responded to this cue. For example, on the previous day, Day 9 postoperatively, as we report in detail in Chapter 3, Mr. James does not resume the conversation because something is not 'right.' As we will see, Mr. James reports, that he was "weirded out" at having been implanted with a machine (BiVAD), a complex situation for patients as we discussed in Chapter 1.

In contrast, today, on Day 10 post-BiVAD implantation, Mr. James does resume the talk and does so by specifying the food he had eaten which elicits in Dr. D the physical sensation of taste: "I could almost taste the turkey sandwich and the fruit cup." The body again! Here Dr. D allows himself to resonate, to receive a message from a physical experience, in this case the pleasure Mr. James is conveying of tasting food. This is important because this experience is anchored in the body, in Dr. D's body. By relating to the experience of tasting food, Dr. D can understand that Mr. James is on the path of recovery from cachexia.

Dr. D's second objective, opening the space for Mr. James to elaborate, provides additional possibilities not only to further the diagnosis, as we just pointed out (first objective), but also to offer Mr. James *a sense* of what is important, creating a sense of 'something that could be there', a possible path towards recovery to engage in. Dr. D does not tell Mr. James this 'something' because Mr. James already knows the list of things he should do (eat, walk, etc.) in order to recover and go home. The issue here is that for Mr. James, lost in the land of dissimilitude, there is no direct correspondence between a list of steps to take and actually taking them. It requires a transformation. This transformation, as we discussed in Chapter 1, is for Mr. James to do. This transformation can only be operated by Mr. James. It involves making sense, on his own terms, of his disease, of how to get out of bed, of how to step on the scale, of how to sit, of how to walk, of how to live his life with the machine, "his" *personal* life. Mr. James needs to elaborate on his own world, his own context, take charge of his life, make sense in his own life. Dr. D provides the safe space for transformation toward *agency* to unfold as Mr. James explores these steps in the process of owning them. We call this the *authenticity of decision* aspect of the encounter.

With this in mind, Mr. James' response is even more exciting for Dr. D because the way Mr. James describes his food *corresponds* to what Dr. D knows to be a description of food by a person who is reversing cachexia. It is followed by Mr. James' evaluation of his feet feeling better and his perspective, his hope, to walk later that same day. Both Mr. James and Dr. D regard this assessment as important: a transformation unfolding. The five seconds of silence (line 10) represent the time that Dr. D is taking to feel and process the experience and to arrive at the insight that Mr. James is taking steps to own his recovery. It is summarized in line 11: "That's good news" and communicated to Mr. James who agrees: "Yes it is" (Line 12). A transformation unfolding because Dr. D and Mr. James recognize and relate to the same 'path.' They are now in synchrony.

When Mr. James adds that the pain is getting better, that he is really looking forward to his physical activity, hoping it will be possible to walk later in the day (line 13), Dr. D's response is:

Beautiful! (line 14)

'Beautiful' appears again, here as it did in Chapter 1 upon learning about the twenty-minute shower taken by Mr. Rice: 'after much trial and error... I took a shower! A twenty-minute long shower!'

'Beautiful!'

A transformation: *selva oscura* (Inferno, Canto I) in *selva antica* (Purgatorio, Canto XVII).

One could say that we are over-interpreting ten lines of a common conversation. Let's see then what happens if we do not do so in the following three possible realities, variations of the same scenario:

Later that day, Mr. James experiences more pain and will neither go for a walk nor get out of bed. It is now ten days after the surgery and several healthcare team members are concerned.

> Scenario 1. Mr. James is lying in bed. A healthcare professional, part of the team, enters the room and realizes that Mr. James is doing none of the regimen steps: Are you sure that the pain is that bad? Oh, come on, you are on Vicodin. You can't be in such pain! If you do not get out of bed, do not walk, you are not helping us support you to a full recovery.
> Mr. James is upset: 'I was told I was lying.'

> Scenario 2. A healthcare professional, part of the team, enters the room. Mr. James is lying in bed. The healthcare professional is worried because Mr. James is neither getting out of bed nor walking nor weighing himself. The healthcare professional now sits down next to Mr. James' bed and asks him what is going on: 'I am in pain,' Mr. James says, 'I have awful pain in my legs, I cannot walk. I have too much fluid in my legs. It is too painful, I really cannot walk.' In a kind voice, the healthcare professional says, 'I understand you are in pain, but you are a young man and it is very important that you weigh yourself every morning and walk to get ready for the transplant. You need to help us help you to recovery.'
> Mr. James is upset: 'They don't believe me. They think I am lying about the pain.'

Understanding that accusing a patient of 'lying' is disrespectful in the professional environment of a hospital, together with additional practice in communication skills turns Scenario 1 into Scenario 2. Yet, the outcome is the same: 'They don't believe me. They think I am lying about the pain.'

> Scenario 3. The healthcare professional thinks that, after all, it is ultimately Mr. James' decision whether he gets out of bed or not. We must respect the patient's decision. If he doesn't want to get out of bed so be it . . . but it will not look good regarding his compliance, cooperation and adherence towards the goal of heart transplantation . . . or maybe Mr. James doesn't really want the transplant. Mr. James is not told that several members of the team think he is exaggerating or even lying about having pain. The team does not trust him.

The consequences of all three scenarios can be ghastly, from a complete withdrawal from participation in his care, to what really happened in Mr. James' case: an escalation of events that prompted the attending physician Dr. D to call for an emergency meeting between patient and team members on Day 12 to address and resolve a very tense situation; Mr. James, before the team meeting, declared he was "preparing for warfare with the team".

"They think I am lying and they do not listen!"

Referring to other team members as "they" as in "they don't listen" or "they think I am lying," can tell us that Mr. James and the attending physician have created a space in which Mr. James feels comfortable talking about the issue; it also tells us that, unfortunately, this person with advanced heart failure, who has gone through such an ordeal — lethal arrhythmias, coding, resuscitations, BiVAD implantation as bridge to heart transplantation — and who now needs to make a full recovery before discharge and before reactivation on the high urgency transplant waiting list, is "preparing for warfare!" There is something fundamentally wrong here.

With or without saying the word "lie", the healthcare professional(s') interpretation of Mr. James' behavior may be summarized as having breached an agreement that was reached on the best course of action for his recovery. The patient agreed to get out of bed each day, walk as much as possible, eat and weigh himself. But, Mr. James is not honoring that agreement. He has unilaterally violated the contract, hence the verdict. All these scenarios presuppose that an agreement has been reached, which indeed it was. A decision had been made and there are expectations from the team and responsibilities allocated to Mr. James to adhere to it and execute its action items.

Such an approach emerges from the normatives regulating a logic of choice (Mol, 2008). Everybody is autonomous[2] and ultimately responsible and accountable for the consequences of their decision (O'Neill, 2002). In the framework of shared decision-making (Dy & Purnell, 2012), the burden of the decision is shared among all stakeholders involved — patient, family and healthcare professionals — working together (Charles, Gafni, & Whelan, 1997). Each stakeholder brings a complementary but necessary perspective to decision support (Elwyn et al., 2010). The framework of shared decision is proposed for the care of advanced heart failure patients (Allen, et al., 2012). Patient, family and healthcare professionals, all of

---

[2]Our RelationalAct concept of patient autonomy is aligned with feminist critique of the concept of autonomy, in which the attributes of the autonomous individual are linked to essentially male values of independence, self-sufficiency and separation from others, neglecting female values of dependence and care (Mackenzie & Stoljar, 2000).

whom have very different knowledge and expectations of the experience of recovery must work together and negotiate the consensus required to make sure that the ensuing actions can and will be in concordance. Ultimately, a consensus is reached, decisions are made and required actions are listed. They come with responsibilities and expectations to adhere to the course of action and treatment. If the agreement is breached, as it is perceived to be by some members of the team in Mr. James' case, guilt appears and it is allocated to the patient: 'You do not help us help you to recovery'. Or worse, abandonment: 'There are "consequences to your behavior".[3] 'You are on your own' and ultimately the benefit of listing the patient for heart transplantation is questioned. This is a dangerous road to travel.

The first obstacle we encounter on this road is the assumption that making a decision and acting upon it are equivalent. However, *'doing it'* requires a *transformation* of 'it' — the decisions, the ideas — into actions, words into action; this transformation as we discussed, is even more complex in the land of dissimilitude. There, a patient is left with the lonely task of transforming the shared-care plan into action with his/her body now in the action, *doing*. This is a body with the specific physiological constraints and manifestations of the advanced heart failure syndrome, and the demands imposed by the critical integration of technological advances, as is the BIVAD, into Mr. James' body. In Chapter 1, with the help of Dante's work, we pointed to the destitution and insolvency of an isolated rational mind organized to make right choices; a mind unable by itself to define its whereabouts, unable to comprehend the reality around it or to continue the journey of the person in the here and now. In *medias res*, the appearance of the light of the rational solution does not serve the purpose of finding the way out. So, how to continue?

Let's go in, there is a meeting going on in Mr. James' room!

Mr. James is sitting up in his bed, looking purposeful and commanding as if towering over both the healthcare team members sitting in the chairs and those standing. Dr. D stands next to Mr. James, waits until everybody is in the room and then opens the meeting. He has the authority to do so. Dr. D

---

[3]Waiting Room. By Monaco, V., and Davis, J. H. Dir. Davis, J. H. The Ronald Reagan UCLA Medical Center, Los Angeles. May 03, 2012. Performance. www.relational medicinefoundation.org.

talks to Mr. James and to him alone. When Dr. D stops, Mr. James will be the one to continue the meeting. The message is clear. Dr. D sits down, closes his eyes and, as he recounts: "and now I shut up". Mr. James takes over, asking the other team members to share their perspectives. Mr. James is in command, Dr. D next to him, listening quietly, his eyes closed; nobody can make eye contact with Dr. D, nobody from the team can form an alliance with him that excludes Mr. James. Everybody listens to Mr. James now. And they do. Dr. D is there, next to Mr. James; Mr. James knows he is there. If something goes wrong, Dr. D will support him, but Dr. D's eyes are closed, no alliances between Mr. James and Dr. D can form to interfere in Mr. James' interaction with the team and exclude the team. Mr. James needs the support of the entire team for the transformation to occur, to regain power over himself, over his life. The team members share their perspectives. Mr. James tells his story connecting his to theirs, translating what their perspectives mean to him. The message is clear: we start from Mr. James' perspective. Dr. D is not opening his eyes, is not saying anything. There is no need to add anything.

The message is clear: the starting point is the patient's perspective, not the algorithm-based perspective abstracting from the patient's perspective and jumping to a shortcut of an immediate translation of average population-based statistical phenotype level symptoms into a mechanistic explanation which would go like this:

> PATIENT: I cannot walk because I have pain in my legs. I think I have too much fluid in the legs when I stand up, it rushes down and my feet swell even more.
> DOCTOR: Hmm fluid retention? Let us see how much is your weight … Oh no, you did not weigh yourself, we cannot verify your claim of fluid overload this way.
> Let us examine your legs then. There is no apparent fluid overload here. Maybe the pain is related to gout.
> Let's test the uric acid, what is the level?
> *And Dante guided by such wisdom turns toward the flickering light of the laboratory: "Uhmm, they are testing my blood. They will know all about me, right down to my genes! I wait here. I wait for them to tell me who I am!"*
> Normal uric acid level, no gout. You do not have pain!
> PATIENT: But I do!
> DOCTOR: Maybe he is faking the pain because he wants more Vicodin …

Oh! We are back in Scenarios 1 to 3! No, let's not start all over again. The meeting has already taken place. We know now we must start from what Mr. James is telling us.

Irreducibility of the Person's Experience

Taking what he says as the irreducible starting point, means that the first question we pose cannot be 'what is the cause of this pain?' This is a subsequent question because it is concerned with natural functions, and explanation of natural processes and functions, and not with the role they play in the person's coping with advanced heart failure — Heidegger (1927/1962) defines the difference and the relation between *presence-at-hand* and *unready-to-hand* (pp. 72–74/102–103). Posing it now would take away the focus from the person, Mr. James, coping with a life with a machine. His body, as a malfunctioning and incomplete organ in need to be attached to a machine, is *obtrusive* (*aufdringlich*, ibid., pp. 73/103). Mr. James is trying to make sense of having his body attached to a machine, his life depending on the machine pumping his heart. He needs to make sense of his life, he needs to see how all this enters *his life*. Only if he can make sense of the machine in his *personal* life, can he integrate it, transcending the 'machine as a foreign body'. If he cannot make sense of the machine in his *personal* life, it remains *obstinate* (*aufsässig*, ibid., pp. 74/103), so much so that he cannot see anything else, cannot see his own life but a life run by a machine.

Helping Mr. James. Yes, the first question is 'how can I help Mr. James?' To be able to really help him, we need to recognize a second obstacle on the road, the *tabula rasa* assumption in the economy of choice. Making a decision, making a choice is not a final point of arrival from which a new beginning, a fresh point of departure emerges from scratch. Rather, it is a process *in medias res*. It is a process that extends and takes place in the continuous transformation of words, ideas and desires, into actions. It is in the action of getting out of bed, walking to the scale, it is *in doing* that the fluid 'rushes to my feet and I feel pain. It is here, in this action that I need help'. The first step is: 'I need you to believe I am in pain even if you do not have an explanation for it'.

This apparently simple step is one of the most difficult to take because it requires both the understanding that our experience is finite and an act of trust. This is not the trust we build because somebody has shown us that s/he can be trusted. This is a trust that can emerge if there is *a priori* understanding and acceptance that the experience of the Other is not 100% known and knowable to us, no matter how large the evidence-based knowledge is, how many laboratory tests we have and continue to perform. If we accept that we do not and cannot know/understand the other person *completely*, we can accept what the Other is saying as essential.[4] We refer to this concept henceforth as *the mystery of the Other*.

Being trained in medicine and doing research in the evidence-based paradigm, the healthcare professional in the encounter with the individual patient is faced with the challenge of translating probabilistic outcome perspectives into the uncertainty of predictions for *this* patient in *this* particular encounter, grounded in the uniqueness of this patient's life.[5] In CoGen Dr. D reflects: If I think that this patient in this encounter is a representative of a group of patients who were part of a randomized clinical trial then I say to myself sentences such as 'this patient fits exactly the criteria of this patient population, therefore he will benefit from this proposed diagnostic or therapeutic intervention (i.e., x dose of Vicodin for pain as in Mr. James' case)'. Only if I transcend this abstraction and consider this patient during this encounter as an individual person (with his/her mystery), can I then say to myself that 'while this patient fulfills the

---

[4]The constitution of self in the encounter with the Other is a strong and central theme in the works of the philosophers Emanuel Levinas and Martin Buber.

[5]The transition that a doctor must make is difficult if we consider Heidegger's interpretation of culture in which scientific inquiry takes place. As we discussed in Chapter 1, what is taken into consideration, what can be studied in science is what Heidegger calls *present-at-hand* (i.e., something's property and its natural functions). It is something that has been stripped out of what its role is, its use in the person's relation to the world, (the *ready-to-hand*.) See Hubert Dreyfus's work (1991) for a clear and rich elaboration of this and other concepts from Division 1 of Heidegger's *Being and Time*. Here we report a passage from Heidegger's *Being and Time* where this is discussed using the example of a tool, a hammer: "When we are using a tool circumspectively, we can say, for instance that the hammer is too heavy or too light. Even the proposition that the hammer is heavy can give expression to a concernful deliberation, and signify that the hammer is not an easy tool — in other words, that it takes force to handle it, or that it will be hard to manipulate. But this proposition *can* also mean that the entity before us, which we know already circumspectively as a hammer, has a weight — that is to say it has a 'property' of heaviness: it exerts a pressure on what lies beneath it, and it falls if this is removed. When this talk is so understood it is no longer spoken with the horizon of awaiting and retaining an equipmental totality and its involvement-relationships. What is said has been grown from looking at what is suitable for an entity with mass" (p. 360–361/412). The equipmental totality and its involvement-relationships are what we in Chapter 1 described as those web of meaningful relations (*significance*) that make our lives familiar.

clinical criteria of the patient group which benefitted from the therapeutic intervention, and is therefore *likely* to benefit from it, this is an individual person and therefore there is no certainty. This is only one step.'

Resonating with the experience of being lost in the land of dissimilitude; estranged from what is known; finding ourselves in the place where all we had known, all which had meaning, has collapsed; no longer being able to make sense of it, to relate to it; we are, as Heidegger argues, at the frontier with death where 'nothing is'. Every step, every turn, every thought is to be relearned. Every day, again, in that corridor, in that boundary layer, what had lost meaning is now reformulating; a tiny messy boundary, where instabilities and small eddies are welcomed and necessary for me to continue to exist. Even pain has to be reintegrated in this unknown context.

Today Mr. James wakes up: "click clack click clack", today somehow, it is louder. Do I need an explanation? I need you to help me relate to the machine, to myself, part man, part machine, do not tell me there is no mechanical malfunctioning and therefore it is not louder than yesterday. Help me make it less loud *and* help me deal with it!

Mr. James, as we see in Chapter 3, needed *both*, more diuretics (as Dr. D had prescribed the day before taking seriously what Mr. James said about his pain in his leg — see line 90, Day 9 post-BiVAD implantation, Chapter 3) *and* help in making his pain less *conspicuous* to make possible a transformation.

No straight line to exit the forest, but a transformation of the collapsed world unrecognizable to me (*selva oscura*) into a world that I recognize to be *familiar to me* (*selva antica*) because anything to which I relate has importance, meaning, necessity, place in *my life*. Every step creates a new opportunity, a new need for transformation. Every step requires an adaptation of a decision on my part, in interaction with the world around me, as a recursive process that changes in time. It is an oscillatory process between the past and present, between the ever-changing conditions including the burden of 'pain in my legs today' and the longing for owning the future, the way I walk, sit, talk, take a shower, live.

Mr. Alcman: I was scared to get out of the room. I just wouldn't. With this thing [LVAD] I didn't know, I couldn't just walk out the room. No. I couldn't.

Mrs. Alcman: Every day, I would go under the door's frame and call him to me: come, come Homer. One step, come!

Mrs. Alcman opens her arms toward him. She smiles, calling his name.

Mr. Alcman: I wouldn't and then, I did. I took one step from the bed, another step toward her. I walked out of the room. I walked out of the building and when I smelled the fresh air I could not take enough, I wanted to walk out all the time.

Mr. Alcman trusts Mrs. Alcman that walking is possible from the bed to the door, with this 'thing', the machine, half in half out of his body; now his body. From his perspective it is impossible. Her calling for him to come to her, to move one step, one only, slowly, makes it possible. And now he walks to her. Only now he can. A transformation unfolds when Mr. Alcman recognizes and relates to the path opened by Mrs. Alcman. This is the synchronization between two persons that we call *dyadism*.

There was no Mrs. Alcman for Mr. James.

Mr. James and his parents are creating paths together. Mr. James from his BiVAD implantation, his parents, struggling with addiction, creating a path for themselves to help Mr. James, as Dr. D learns more from Mr. James on Day 21 post-BiVAD implantation:

Day 21 post-BiVAD implantation

83	Mr. James:	Something that is helping me cope um with
84		in here is this book I've got here.
85		Believe it or not I've gotten a lot from it.
86		It's for uh dealing with alcoholics and addicts,
87		but it's also helping me get insight on other aspects in life
88		and you know
89		it really definitely
90		uh transcends to more than one area of my life and other areas,
91		it's definitely a good book.
92		I recommend it even if
93		you are not dealing with the stress of a family member, friend
94		that is struggling with addiction when you read.
95		I mean it's just a helpful, very helpful book.

Mr. and Mrs. Alcman's experiences are not the same as those of Mr. James and his parents. Not more/less difficult, not more/less dramatic, they are incommensurable. Each patient, a different story, different victories and struggles, unique *mysteries*. The transformations, as Mr. and Mrs. Alcman and Mr. James and his parents know, are not done alone but with the help of the Other. While alone, lost in the land of dissimilitude, one is not isolated and can transform the *selva oscura* into *selva antica*.

Are the transformation processes happening in the interactions between doctor and patient? If so, how do they look?

Temporality

To answer these questions, we resume our encounter with Dr. D and Mr. James on Day 10 postoperatively, just a minute after we left them.

Dr. D and Mr. James have just finished talking about Mr. James' parents, and Dr. D is remarking on their engagement in supporting Mr. James (line 45–49).

Then Dr. D recuperates[6] Mr. James' past and future not only as temporal events that already happened and that will be happening, but as those relations that Mr. James has built in his life with his parents:

Day 10 post-BiVAD implantation

45	Dr. D:	And I saw both your parents are really good.
46	Mr. James:	Yeah.
47	Dr. D:	They are concerned,
48		very involved, very proactive,
49		ready to do anything that needs to be done.
50	Mr. James:	Yea.
51		And I think my uncle is coming out next week so.
52	Dr. D:	And I liked the way they talked about Uncle M you know?
53	Mr. James:	Yea. Yea. He's a great guy. He's a great guy.
54	Dr. D:	Yea.
55	Mr. James:	So.
56	Dr. D:	Yea, so that's great so um they have the homework of looking
57		for [a place].
58	Mr. James:	[a place] to stay. Yea.
59	Dr. D:	And the teaching,
60	Mr. James:	teaching of the BIVAD and all of that,
61	Dr. D:	and then

On line 56, Dr. D refers to Mr. James' parents looking for a place to live with Mr. James. This is as per safety protocol, for the first three months following the mechanical assist device implantation, Mr. James and his family must temporarily relocate to a place within a one-hour driving distance from the hospital. Dr. D also *recuperates* activities that

---

[6]We use the term 'recuperate' as a move to recruit past and future into present to help Mr. James. In this sense it is not just a recapitulation/summary of a list of activities done or to be done, but a retrieval of images, history and activities needed to help Mr. James.

Mr. James does with his parents: BiVAD teaching on line 60 refers to *VAD teaching* session in which Mr. James and his parents learn to live with the BiVAD, i.e., how to take a shower with the shower kit, how to change the bandage of the BiVAD without infecting the entrance wound where the cable reaches out to the battery and computer set (the controller as shown in Figure 2.1), fundamental tasks all patients with implanted assist devices and their families caring for them must learn. These are activities that Mr. James is doing together with his parents. In participating in these activities, Mr. James is involved with those who care for him and are important to him in his life, in a way that defines who he is. These relations, that Mr. James has built in his life with his parents, are rooted in his past and create a potential for his future, that is actuated in every moment to moment in his present. The transformation of his present needs a sense of his own past and future as constitutive components from which to emerge (Raia & Deng, 2011). Let's consider for example, a relation with a loved one. This person has been part of one's life (past) and this person is also part of one's future; what one does, dreams, builds now is based also on having this person in one's life — past and future here not linearly related in a sequence of events. If the death of the loved one occurs then a person's possibilities for the future, as it has been built on the relation with the loved one alive, changes and one makes sense of life in the here and now differently.

We have been introducing the participating patients in this study by giving a brief description of: their relations to others, what they do and/or what they like to do (e.g., mother, father, wife, husband, son, friend, nurse, subway conductor, lawyer, writer) because these as identities represent constitutive relations in a person's biographical historicity. In *Being and Time* (p. 143/182), Heidegger discusses how intertwined these two ways of making sense are: one of dealing with things in the world(s), and the other making sense of who one is as a person with others, as a son, as a doctor, as a patient (identities). Mr. James is making sense of how to survive with a BiVAD by learning how to change the battery of a BiVAD with his parents. In these activities, the machine becomes slowly interconnected with the involvement-relationship in Mr. James' world (his family, his temporal being in the past-future). The machine becomes slowly familiar for him and his body. He is no longer feeling only the being-tethered-to-a-machine, he can do other things in his life, with his family and friends, in his work, integrating an identity of being a person with advanced heart failure in his life. From learning to survive using a BiVAD, he is learning to live his life with the BiVAD. The BiVAD now is acquiring a role in the activities Mr. James is engaged in. As we discussed in Chapter 1, it has become *significant*: meaningfully webbed in his life.

As we have discussed, a person is engaged in the world acting and relating to things transparently (Heidegger, 1927/1962). For example, sitting in a chair was for Mr. Montale before the LVAD implantation (Chapter 1) done without thinking about sitting, or about how tall the chair was, as the chair was simply a *ready-to-hand* tool for use. Mr. Montale simply sat on it to have a delicious meal with his wife. The activity was part of his identity as a husband. When things as one's own body become obtrusive and a sense of who we are is broken and becomes unrecognizable, one is in the *selva oscura*. As we discuss in Chapter 1, Heidegger says that there we are alone. Yes we are. It is true, we cannot understand the *selva oscura*, or be in the land of dissimilitude through the experience of another person living it. However, high-tech advances are forcing us into territories we did not explore before. In the practice of high-tech modern medicine, as we see it here enacted in advanced heart failure, one cannot go through the land of dissimilitude alone. It is in this practice that we see how it is possible to recognize and help somebody in the *selva oscura:* When all that is familiar has broken down, the patient needs help to start coping with things in the world in his/her own way, redevelop a *significance* in the world, a familiarity with it, and by doing so, start making sense of his/her life, of his/her identity. It is this act in high-tech modern medicine that is a Relational*Act*.

In Mr. James' room, Dr. D recruits Mr. James' past and future into his present action and activities with his parents, so as to help Mr. James elaborate the experience of living with a BiVAD as his own. Dr. D then introduces actions to be taken (from line 61 onwards) so that Mr. James can start recognizing them on his path (lines 64, 67–68).

62	Dr. D:	and then
63		all the discharge planning between [Dates removed]
64		and then waiting list
65	Mr. James:	Sounds good.
66	Dr. D:	heart transplant and two weeks later

67		a happy life for the next hundred years.
68	Mr. James:	Sounds good.
69		Sounds great!
70	Dr. D:	With all these rules coming in for the biopsies,
71		but you will have no problem doing it.
72	Mr. James:	Probably not.
73		Definitely no problem there.
74		And then after I'm done recovering,
75		I go up to Alaska.
76		Be ready for me to bring you a lot of fish.

The BiVAD attached to his body, so *obstinate* (*aufsässig*, Heidegger, 1927/1962), can start becoming part of Mr. James' life. In this involvement-relationship in Mr. James' world, the BiVAD being attached to his body does not take charge of his life. In other words, Mr. James will be discharged with an implanted BiVAD and not the BiVAD discharged with Mr. James attached to it.

In recognizing a path, a horizon for himself, Mr. James has a sense of who he is and can start transforming his present.

When Mr. James refers to Alaska (lines 74–75), he is already in the process of transformation of the present as Mr. Alcman was in taking his steps toward Mrs. Alcman.

We can meet Dante again. Out of the tenebrous *Inferno* where time is annihilated in the eternity of the constant darkness of a static past, we meet again in *Purgatorio*. Here, there is an essential retrieval of time. Dante here meets those who billow between the memory of the past unfolding as relational acts and the certainty of salvation, between past (memory) and hope, possibilities (future).

Attunement and Synchronization

In order to support Mr. James in this transformation, Dr. D must be able to recognize a person in the land of dissimilitude and learn specifically how to relate to this person. For Dr. D, this means learning from Mr. James about his life and attuning to how high-tech modern medicine is appearing to Mr. James: his BiVAD implantation, his staying in hospital, his experience of *obtrusiveness*, his body with the BiVAD attached.

Attunement is a process that builds in time. We know that so far Dr. D and Mr. James met each day for the last 10 days. They learned about the Other and, as we already anticipated, Dr. D can now tell when Mr. James is being quieter than usual, indicating that he is going through some difficulties. This is a recursive process that we call *iteration aspect of the encounter*.

It is not a linear process of adding new information and new knowledge. It is a process that is embedded in the specific situation of the medical encounter, as it cannot be independent from the relational aspects on which it builds.

While in the long-term, attunement to the Other develops, Dr. D responds to the specific situation with Mr. James as he was building on the moment-by-moment interactions in the encounter with Mrs. More (as seen in the Introduction).

Day 10 post-BiVAD implantation

76	Dr. D:	I'd like that. (2.0 s)
77		When my wife and I um
78		we just came over a year ago from [City name].
79	Mr. James:	Yeah.
80	Dr. D:	And um we had ...
81		she's from [Country] and I'm originally from [Country].
82	Mr. James:	Yeah.
83	Dr. D:	So when we had uh,
84		she was a professor in [University name] and
85		I was at [University name]
86		so we thought we would be there for a lifetime
87		and four years ago um we bought this little place
88		in the [geographical name]
89		on a little trout stream
90	Mr. James:	Whoow.
91	Dr. D:	So we learned fly fishing
92		and now then we are here
93		and so since that's our soul place
94		we said we are not selling it
95		and we were just renting it you know?
96	Mr. James:	Yeah.
97	Dr. D:	It is a beautiful place
98		in the woods.
99	Mr. James:	Oh yeah.
100	Dr. D:	And you can do a morning sun salute.
101		In this beautiful nature
102		... so it's good to have a soul place.
103	Mr. James:	YES!
104		Yes
105		I think Alaska is where my soul is.
106	Dr. D:	I can see that.
107		I feel it in the way you say it.

Dr. D perceives that Alaska is not just a fishing spot for Mr. James. It is offered as a beautiful vision, something to look forward to, as soon as Mr. James recovers. It is a soul place, as Mr. James confirms at lines 103–104. Dr. D resonates with it and shares with Mr. James his own soul place (lines 77–102). Note that Dr. D is sharing what for him is important. The places (we removed the names of cities, countries of origin and universities), from which he and his wife come, where they worked and lived, creating a new home far from the countries of origin; a life's journey. The forms are different — poetry in one case and high-tech modern medicine encounter talk in the other — but Virgil's encounter with Dante in Canto I and Dr. D's encounter with Mr. James, resonating on a soul place, are similar: a person's life journey from the place of birth to the place where a person develops his/her own *personal* life.

Rispousemi: " non omo, omo già fui,	"Not man; although I was a man," he replied
e li parenti miei furon lomabrdi,	69 "My parents were both Mantuans. I descend
mantoani per patrïa ambedui.	from those of Lombardy on either side.
Nacqui sub Iulio, ancor che fosse tardi,	I was born *sub Julio*, at the latter end.
e vissi a Roma sotto 'l buon Augusto	72 Under the good Augustus I lived at Rome,
nel tempo de li dei falsi e bugiardi.	in the days when false and lying gods
	still reigned.
Poeta fui e cantai di quell giusto	I was a poet, and I sang of him,
figliuol d'Anchise che venne di Troia,	75 Anchises's righteous son, who sailed
	from Troy
poi che 'l superbo Iïón fu combusto.	after the burning of proud Ilium.
Ma perché tu ritorni a tanta noia?	But why do you turn back toward trouble?

Interestingly, it is Dante, the writer, who chooses how Virgil, his guide through the land of dissimilitude, can introduce himself to Dante, the pilgrim: through a person's journey. In high-tech modern medicine, a process of attuning happens. At lines 74–75 Mr. James names Alaska and Dr. D replies immediately with two seconds of silence following.

Living with advanced heart failure always presupposes an unpredictable winding road ahead; to give a patient the best chances to have a good outcome, Dr. D feels it is important to create a stable bond, a bond that is based on a personal sharing of one's own personal journey. Sharing a soul place, is a strong candidate theme for getting this goal accomplished: a dyadic encounter where there is a moment for resonating with something that both Mr. James and Dr. D consider to be an important part of their lives. This is important as it enables Dr. D to maintain the vision of a soul place floating in Mr. James' room, as a real possibility for Mr. James. The attunement emerging from the sharing of a soul place opens as a horizon for Mr. James' life. The resonating with a soul place as the past and the possibilities of the future after transplantation creates a path for Mr. James in the present to take the next steps towards recovery, leaving the hospital and then undergoing heart transplantation after which Alaska is finally reachable. It is a subtle process, as a real sharing of soul places must be. As we make sense of Dr. D's resonating with Mr. James' image/possibilities of going to Alaska after his recovery and bringing a lot of fish (lines 73–75), Emanuel Levinas's concept of intersubjective responsibility (Levinas, 1979) can be helpful as Dr. D responds to an imperative to care.

It cannot be a didactic move: 'if you walk and adhere to the regimen, you will be able to go to Alaska'; or worse, a move to maintain power over a patient: 'we will see, when you will feel better, let's not get ahead of ourselves'; as both approaches prevent a person in the here and now to assume *agency* in their own recovery and recognize their life as their own.

The sharing does not translate into Dr. D becoming emotionally vulnerable as a doctor, as resonating on a human experience still maintains the specificity of Dr. D's and Mr. James' own experiences. Yet, sharing those important things that can resonate with another person's life, has a *function* in the medical encounter of high-tech modern medicine, to care for a patient: to guide integration of treatments, goals and technological advancement into *this specific person's* life.

'To care' is a complex *process*. It emerges in the dynamics of interactions with the Other. It requires a continuous *attunement* with short-term moment-to-moment *synchronization* to the Other and to the dynamic situation of the encounter. As such, it is open to rupture and requires continuous re-synchronization.

A few moments later in the medical encounter with Mr. James, this process of rupture and re-synchronization occurs.

Day 10 post-BiVAD implantation

108	Mr. James:	I strongly recommend
109		you to get up there one of these days
110		and do some good fishing.
111		(2.0 s)
112	Dr. D:	Mmm hmm I think that's a good idea.
113	Mr. James:	Yes, very much so.
114		(2.0 s)
115	Dr. D:	Good idea!
116	Mr. James:	Very much so!

In CoGen, listening to this passage, Dr. D recoiled from the table on which the taped encounter was playing, and shared his first reactions to this short exchange transcribed on lines 108–110: " 'I strongly recommend' is a very directing way of talking, I mean it's the patient sitting there and . . . you know the classical role distribution would be I'm the one who does recommend things."

So, Dr. D's immediate reaction was to recoil from this situation as he perceived there was a prospect of role change, where Mr. James takes charge and deference to the doctor's function to guide the patient is forgotten: a challenge of authority. Dr. D's first reaction had the power to taint his response in the medical encounter. Two seconds of silence (line 111). Dr. D's actual response is flat and non-committal; it has a closing flair to it.

His reaction should not come as surprise; as we discuss above, synchronization is a process and not a state; the understanding of the doctor's role and his function is a process in the practice of medicine that needs continuous attuning to the Other, to the specific situation and to the understanding of the doctor's own role to be a guide to integrate treatments, goals and technological advancements in medicine for *this patient* in *this situation*. For the two seconds of silence (line 111), Dr. D describes it in CoGen as "something was not right" and recalls "wait a minute . . . how do I feel about going fishing there after just having talked about a ventricular assist device and heart transplantation for him? It's a rapid transition into something else. I need to go through my own identity in that moment, who am I in that encounter? And then I realize, I have been claiming that I'm in the encounter as a person. So I need to allow myself for real to just be a person. A radically naked person, you know, just a *person*." A person, going fishing in a soul place. This image of a doctor's thinking of his patient having gone through BiVAD, then the transplantation, and finally in Alaska, fishing in his soul place, inviting his 'doc': 'that' Dr. D says: "is as good as things can get." Good idea!

If synchronization does not take place, there are three possible responses to Mr. James' charge. One is to ignore it, for example starting the physical examination: "let me listen to you" missing the opportunity to utilize the therapeutic power of encouraging a patient to think about, to desire, to visualize what a patient loves and can do after transplantation, living his/her own life out of the hospital. In Mr. James' case, it is thinking about his going to Alaska, his soul place, fishing. A second possibility is to say: "Okay let's see how you do after transplant." That is, Mr. James, don't go overboard with your personhood, let's first see if you're still alive after transplantation. Don't get too excited about things. A very discouraging message. The third possibility is to think to oneself and say to the patient: "Okay let's not talk about fishing right now, we have to first get you through this", another discouraging type of response rescinding any possible connection to life outside the hospital.

Re-examining one's personal narratives allows learning to care. The patient's journey to re-establishing and re-constituting his/her own identity is also a process experienced by the doctor re-defining her/his professional identity in the attunement of the dyadic encounter.

CHAPTER 3
THE RELATIONAL*ACT*

We shadow Dr. D in Mr. James' room. We follow one of their encounters from beginning to end and reflect on it as we have done in CoGen sessions. It is Day 9 post-BiVAD operation.

1	Dr. D:	Hello young man!
2		How is life?
3	Mr. James:	I'm fine.

Silence.

Mr. James is lying in bed, a high-tech hospital bed with all the electrical controls to move the body, up the head, down the feet, rock to side. The hospital gown is opened in the front revealing a 10 inch-long (~25 cm) wound from the incision that was made down the sternum to spread the ribs apart and access the heart area. Stitches keep it closed now; it is dark yellow-brown and long. All around it, overboarding the hospital gown, electrical cables connect electrodes to the EKG recorder. The heart's activity is displayed on a black monitor showing a green line, the heart rate.

Silence. "Click clack click clack."

5	Dr. D:	So, on Friday a week ago when it came up,
6		Friday morning was when we said let's do
7		the high emergency status for heart transplantation listing
8		and maybe we have an organ coming up during the weekend.
9		That was also when we first met.
10	Mr. James:	Yah.
11	Dr. D:	and then we said okay and Dr. Hort[1] was already a little skeptical
12		and said maybe if anything happens we have to go ahead.
13		And this was in the night
14		and so then it was clear
15		we have to recommend the Bi-Ventricular Assist Device.

---

[1]Dr. Hort was the attending physician when Mr. James was hospitalized. Dr. Hort was on service until the day before Mr. James' BiVAD implantation when Dr. D started his two weeks service.

CoGen session:
Federica (Researcher): Let's listen to this again.

1	Dr. D:	*Hello young man!*
2		*How is life?*
3	Mr. James:	*I'm fine.*

Federica: [stops the tape and counts the seconds aloud] 1, 2, 3... long silence. Mario you continue by recalling events that happened a week before — the high emergency status heart transplant listing (line 7), when you first met — just prior to BiVAD implantation. Would you walk me through what is happening?

Mario (Dr. D): When I entered the room, I expected to see Mr. James, a very handsome young man with his long hair looking like Jesus — full of inner life, vision, energy and dignity despite adversity — sitting up in the middle of the bed as if he were holding his two pumps, one on each side.

Federica: Your gesturing of Mr. James' expected position — sitting up straightening your back, extending your arms as if to embrace the machines — gives me an impression of expecting somebody in charge, a victorious young man.

Mario: Yes! Exactly! Having survived major crises, being resuscitated, undergoing a major heart surgery, being extubated on Day 1 postop (postoperatively), sitting in the chair and already having started physical therapy on Day 2 postop, that is immense! What an achievement!

Federica: Yes ...

Mario: Mr. James should be in the same framework of excitement for such progress as I am.

Federica: Is he?

Mario: No, I do not feel it here. He is in bed with his two assist-heart pumps, one on each side, but does not tower over them like a king.

Mario: [punches his right fist into his left hand with a movement that feels like an energetic punch on life]: I can fight!
So when I enter and see him deflated, crouching in the bed that seems now too big for him and he says 'fine' ... in my framework, just 'fine' is not a good sign nine days after a major surgery; just 'fine' does not grasp the immensity of what just happened, of what Mr. James went through.

Federica: He needs energy to fight for the recovery, like your punch [Federica punches her left hand]: I can fight!

Mario: Exactly! The optimal state, not only recovering physically from BiVAD implantation but to achieve the best possible long-term outcome after heart transplantation with *post-transplantation management* goals of (1) maintenance of allograft function, (2) minimization of side effects of immunosuppression drugs, (3) coping with the transplantation process, and (4) complete reintegration into society,[2] he must be best prepared by a full emotional state of being active and taking ownership of his critical condition.

Preparation Phase

One can speculate that in order to process all that we discussed in the above CoGen session in such a short interval of time of the medical encounter (lines 1–4), Dr. D must have information we do not have. And this is quite so.

Before entering Mr. James' or any other patient's room, Dr. D reviews the patient's medical record. In addition, he imagines/visualizes the person he will be meeting and his/her story: What has just happened in this person's life? Is it the first time he is meeting this patient? If not, what is the patient's medical history? If the meeting is in *out*patient clinic, is it a routine visit? If the patient is hospitalized, as is the case for Mr. James, is it right after a major surgery?

Describing his meeting with Mr. James, Dr. D says: "*When I entered the room, I expected to see Mr. James, a very handsome young man with his long hair looking like Jesus — full of inner life, vision, energy and dignity despite adversity — sitting up in the middle of the bed as if he were holding his two pumps, one on each side.*" By visualizing we do not mean creating simply a mental representation of the person he will be meeting. In reality, Dr. D, through anticipation, develops a sense of his expectations. By doing so he makes his expectations available to himself: how the person who had undergone a specific surgical procedure (e.g., an emergency BiVAD implantation as a bridge to transplantation as in the case of Mr. James) and/or is participating in family and work events, (e.g., the person is preparing for the wedding of his/her daughter, or moved back to live with the parents) will look, sit, or talk, as these different experiences have an impact on how a person appears or communicates.

---

[2]The post-transplantation management goals are discussed in Deng (2010).

As we discussed in Chapter 2, based on what he has learned in the recurring medical encounters with a specific patient, the *iteration* aspect of the encounter, Dr. D can envision more details as well as richer and more dynamic images of the person he will meet, as if entering in the middle of that person's life. This is more than a static mental picture. As Dr. D visualizes how the person with whom he is about to meet will move, talk, sit, or say hello in the specific contextual situation of that patient's own medical history and family, work and life events, he is attuning to a *mood*.

Before entering Mr. James' room, Dr. D is envisioning a victorious young man, towering over his pumps, having successfully fought death with the support of the healthcare team. His recovery has been impressively fast; full recovery is closer and Mr. James will finally be reactivated on the transplant list, be transplanted and get the BiVAD off his chest, figuratively and literally. Dr. D has a specific vision of Mr. James' entire clinical course and a sense of where at the present moment Mr. James should be within this larger context. What Dr. D is envisioning is not only a physical appearance in relation to the medical history of the person but also a mood, a way of being he will encounter. This is an important relational aspect as Heidegger (1927/1962) discusses how we are always 'in a mood' not as an inner disposition but as an attunement to our way of being, our life (pp. 134/172). As Dreyfus (1991) discusses, "moods determine not just what we do but how things show up for us" (p. 172). In this framework, Dr. D's anticipation is an attunement to the expected mood in the encounter of the Other.

We call this entire process of preparing for the medical encounter in high-tech modern medicine the *preparation phase*.

Upon entering the room on Day 9, expecting Mr. James towering over his pumps, Dr. D is quick to realize that Mr. James is actually not looking as anticipated. Mr. James, his shoulders hunched, is huddled in a bed that now looks too big for him. To the question: 'How is life?' Mr. James responds: 'I'm fine.' Just 'fine', Dr. D worries.

It is the preparation before the encounter that allows Dr. D, in the subsequent phase of the medical encounter, which we call the *initiation phase*, to contrast the anticipated encounter with the person and the actual encounter.

Initiation Phase

1	Dr. D:	Hello young man!
2		How is life?
3	Mr. James:	I'm fine

} *Initiation Phase*

The question on line 2, as we discussed in Chapter 2, opens up a space for Mr. James to select the preferred topic as the first subject in the medical conversation. This question is a common opening question in Dr. D's medical encounters with his patients.

The patient's answer, Mr. James' answer here, together with his medical and biographical records and the expected/observed[3] (anticipated/experienced) scenario differential, serve as a critical diagnostic tool, assembled at the person level.

Preparing for the medical encounter by both reviewing the information before entering the encounter and anticipating the mood, 'visualizing' the encounter, Dr. D has a framework for comparison based on the most up-to-date clinical information. This enables him to pick up on any discrepancy (or concordance) in the observed (experienced) situation of the encounter and to reliably and rapidly compare expected and observed impression. The expected/observed (anticipated/experienced) comparison can pertain to organ function data, e.g., the skin taking on a yellow color when the liver is failing, or to data integrated on the person level. In Mr. James' case, the person level data used in the *preparation phase* is Mr. James' excellent course of recovery during the first days postoperatively and his loquacious style of communication as seen in Chapter 2. Together, these data form Dr. D's 'visualization' of a young man, victorious over death.

So, when Dr. D contrasts the *initiation phase's* observation of how Mr. James sits in his bed and how Mr. James answers the question 'How is life?' to the *preparation phase's* expectations, the discrepancy alarms him.

The role of expectation in the Relational*Act*

In the same way that the framework of choice/decision-making creates expectation and responsibility as developed in the three scenarios described in Chapter 2, the *preparation phase* in the framework of the Relational*Act* does also create expectations. However, the expectations emerging in the

---

[3]Expected/observed is a classical terminology used in clinical medicine. It has a mere cognitive connotation that we do not wish to endorse. Nevertheless we utilize it as clinicians are familiar with it and can better relate to what we are describing as anticipated/experienced. In the encounter, Dr. D is actually both experiencing and observing, as in the process of attuning (as described in Chapter 2) he can experience the situation at hand, and utilize his experience to assess the situation at the same time. In the model of skills acquisition (Dreyfus & Dreyfus, 2000) adopted by the American Council for Graduate Medical Education (ACGME), this mastery would be an example of Stage 5, Expert.

logic of choice are significantly different from the ones emerging in the *preparation phase* of the Relational*Act*. There are no moral normatives organizing Dr. D's evaluation of Mr. James' appearance, behavior and stance, there is, rather, an imperative for Dr. D to care. This is evident in the way the results of Dr. D's assessment are translated into action. Rather than a verdict on compliance, adherence or cooperation, beginning on line 5, Dr. D recounts and reconstitutes for Mr. James all the steps he has taken thus far, in an integrated cohesive story, a meaningful path unfolding. Estranged from what is recognized, in the place where all which had meaning has collapsed, where it is no longer possible to make sense of things, there, in the land of dissimilitude one is lost but not isolated: Virgil walks with Dante. In Mr. James' room, rather than concentrating on the appearance of isolated symptoms, Dr. D moves to help Mr. James to re-elaborate his journey.

The translation of the assessment, done in the *initiation phase*, into the act of reconstituting for Mr. James all the steps taken on his path into a cohesive story, transitions the encounter into the next phase: the *continuation phase*.

Continuation Phase

5	Dr. D:	So, on Friday a week ago when it came up
6		Friday morning was when we said let's do
7		the high emergency status heart transplantation listing
8		and maybe we have an organ coming up during the weekend
9		That was also when we first met.
10	Mr. James:	Yeah.
11	Dr. D:	And then we said okay and Dr. Hort was already a little skeptical
12		and said maybe if anything happens we have to go ahead.
13		And this was in the night
14		and so then it was clear
15		we have to recommend the Bi-ventricular Assist Device.

In reconstituting for Mr. James the steps taken on his path as a cohesive story, Dr. D can now address what he hypothesizes is one of the sources for the discrepancy in the expected/observed data. Dr. D asks Mr. James to share his experience of illness as integral part of the medical encounter.

The role of the illness experience in the RelationalAct

16	Dr. D:	How did it feel when the question came up on the assist device?
17		You were prepared on Saturday morning,
18		you know on the 12th?
19	Mr. James:	It was it was a little weird, you know,
20		kind of I mean (3.0 s)
21		it's just kind of
22		uh, uh a little trippy uhmm
23		hearing something like you know
24		like that.
25		It weirded me out with the gangliectomy you know
26		you don't wanna do it (2.0 s)
27		but if it's really for the best you kind of wanna do it.
28		But it's just weird to think about it you know. (1.5 s)
29		And uhmm I am glad it's happened you know. (3.0 s)

At line 19, Mr. James starts sharing his experience for the first time. It is an experience of estrangement waking up with the machine as part of one's own body. This experience is shared by other patients as discussed in Chapters 1 and 2 and as Mr. James, a few months later, during an interview, recalls feeling "like a scary character in the movies, half man, half machine."

There are long silences (1.5 to 3 seconds) in Mr. James' talk elaborating his experience. These silences are not interrupted by the physician.

30	Dr. D:	Yeah, yeah.
31		It's a *big* (1.5 s) thing.
32	Mr. James:	Yes! (2.0 s)
33		Very big thing.

Grounded in the understanding, as discussed in Chapter 2, that the Other is not completely known and knowable to us (Levinas, 1979) which we called the *mystery of the Other* aspect of the encounter, Dr. D listens very attentively and accepts what Mr. James is saying as essential. This enables him to realize that there are long silences in Mr. James' talk and that Mr. James searches for words to describe his experience. Dr. D notices also that Mr. James does not name the BiVAD. Specifically, Mr. James refers to it as 'trippy … hearing something, you know, like that' (lines 19–24) and uses the word 'weird' three times (line 19, 25 and 28). It is on this word, 'weird', that Dr. D operates the first transformation, from 'weird' into 'big' (line 31). Note that the pause of 1.5 seconds (line 31) after Dr. D uses the word 'big,' gives space to the word and greater emphasis on the transformation. 'Yes! It is a very big thing', echoes Mr. James (line 33). This is an important operation because 'weird', 'strange', 'freaky' are all terms that imply a 'pushing away', an estrangement from a person, from an object, from a place. 'Big' does not have this connotation and, in this context, can be elaborated as an accomplishment, as transforming something obtrusive into one's personal life. It *is* an accomplishment for Mr. James. Dr. D and Mr. James transform 'trippy' things into big things (e.g., the BiVAD) being accepted in the person's body and life. The illness experience is not just shared and communicated, but utilized to care for the patient. As such, it becomes integral to the medical encounter.

34	Dr. D:	And it was for us,
35		we would have liked to see the heart transplantation at this
36		surgery but at the same time
37		since no one knows how long the waiting time [is]
38	Mr. James:	[Ye]ah.
39	Dr. D:	There was this arrhythmia that that you [had].
40	Mr. James:	[de]finitely.
41	Dr. D:	This was not possible.
42	Mr. James:	I definitely agree that this was the best decision,
43		I am very glad I went along with it (2 s).
44	Dr. D:	Yah (2 s).

Dr. D communicates that the teams shares Mr. James' disappointment (lines 34–35) at having to go through a BiVAD implantation as bridge to transplantation instead of having directly a heart transplantation surgery as a single stage heart replacement.

The role of attuning and synchronization in the RelationalAct

At this time of the *continuation phase* of the Day 9 encounter, we notice an interesting phenomenon: as shown in the bracketed words, Mr. James' talk starts to overlap[4] that of Dr. D.

---

[4]Note that we use the notation: [word]
                                     [word]
with words enclosed in square brackets aligned one beneath the other to denote the start and the end of overlapping talk as it is customary for adjacent lines in conversation analysis (Heritage & Maynard, 2006).

In addition to overlapping Dr. D's talk, Mr. James twice uses the word 'definitely' (lines 40 and 42). From both the overlap talk and the use of the word 'definitely', Dr. D receives the impression that Mr. James wishes to conclude this part of the conversation and move to a different topic. We use the term 'receives the impression' because by listening so attentively to Mr. James, Dr. D is, as Kenneth Tobin puts it, radically listening (Tobin, 2009); that is, Dr. D is not thinking what to say next, nor formulating a response to what Mr. James says, but allowing himself to learn as much as possible from Mr. James. By doing so, Dr. D recovers a pattern: the conspicuous absence of terms such as 'BiVAD' and 'machine' in all that Mr. James has said so far, replaced with the use of the word 'weird' three times (lines 19, 25 and 28).

In the two-second-long silence at line 43, Dr. D elaborates what he has perceived as Mr. James' signals to conclude this part of the conversation and based on this, prepares to move to the next step. "Yah," Dr. D acknowledges, remaining silent for another two seconds, following this conclusion statement at line 44, to be sure that Mr. James has nothing more to add on this topic.

These moments of shared silence are based on the understanding that two persons are communicating and together (*dyadism*) they are ready for the next step. We saw this process unfold in the Introduction, during Dr. D's encounter with Mrs. More in the acceptance of a common understanding of death as part of life, emerging from the visual experience of nodding, the rhythm of Ms. More's nods as a cue for the physician's response; the auditory experience, the length of the sound of silences and the repetition of talk setting up a rhythm.[5]

45	Dr. D:	Okay.
46		Now you know we are in a good position
47		because the plan is clear, so
48		when your parents come a little later
49		we just go through kind of planning getting out of here.
50		And the question when to accept a heart transplant offer
51		becomes the next question.
52	Mr. James:	Yeah.
53	Dr. D:	And usually we wait until,
54		if you are well you know,

---

[5]Please refer to Footnote 7 in Chapter 1 on Heidegger's discussion of communication.

55		your health [is]
56	Mr. James:	[I] had major surgery
57		and its many weeks so I definitely understand the setback there.
58	Dr. D:	A little you know
59		a little time to get well.
60	Mr. James:	Yeah.
61	Dr. D:	The time to get well is vari[able]
62	Mr. James:	[Yes]
63	Dr. D:	[a:nd]
64	Mr. James:	[it va]ries from person to person.

To take the next step (lines 45–52), Dr. D acknowledges where he and Mr. James are (lines 45–47) and opens a path where Mr. James is not alone but with his parents in this process (line 48), a path that as we see in Chapter 2, has relational elements of Mr. James' past and future — an activity to be done with his parents. In creating the space for a possible transformation, Dr. D gives a direction to where they are going (lines 47–52) and making plans (line 47 and 49).

And now, with the possibilities of taking the next steps to prepare for the future heart transplantation, Mr. James acknowledges the setback (line 57) created by the emergency BiVAD implantation.

As Dr. D is learning, while it is important to assess and acknowledge any obstacles on his path to recovery, for Mr. James it is equally important not to dwell on them. He does acknowledge obstacles once he has found a possible way to make changes and has a plan on how to move ahead, and by doing so, he is able to deal and cope with obstacles. Mr. James' mode of dealing with obstacles is not questioned by Dr. D. This is of particular importance as Mr. James does not recognize himself as a person who talks about obstacles without having already a possible way to tackle them. As they are a *dyad*, Dr. D is attuned to Mr. James' talk and talk overlap and moves the conversation beyond the 'setback', initiating another transformation: the 'setback', i.e., the BiVAD implantation as a bridge to transplantation, becomes a step in the process of getting well. The use of the word 'setback' suggests an image of a path with a direction toward recovery. On lines 58–59, Dr. D is transforming the image of moving backward on this linear path into one of being in a recognizable space, an image that suggests a process in time, moving into 'getting well,' and an image that requires actions into what is familiar: getting out of the hospital and going home, it is not a linear path as it requires that an *obtrusive* body attached to an *obstinate*[6] machine transforms into a life out of here. Here, in the hospital, is the place where Mr. James learns to deal with the BiVAD as an equipment, he learns how to use it, how to walk with it and slowly integrate it in his life. This movement from 'BiVAD as a 'setback' to 'we are on the trajectory to recovery and full restitution to a life out of here', provided in a safe space of the medical encounter where Dr. D can assume an holding function,[7] leads to synchronization of perspectives: two persons acting in the same framework, reciprocally relating to one another (*dyadism*). It is in *relating to the Other* that processes of synchronization can emerge. This understanding of *relating-to* we call the Relational*Act*.

65	Dr. D:	Yah. Yah.
66		And you have been
67		since just the very beginning of this doing very well,
68		getting going.
69	Mr. James:	Well I had a lot of encouragement (1.4 s)
70		Doctors like you and the nursing staff
71		makes me want to do better.
72	Dr. D:	Yah (2 s).
73		And the question may come up
74		let's assume after the memorial weekend you can go home.
75		The home near the hospital.[8]
76	Mr. James:	Yeah.
77	Dr. D:	Uhhh that we won't have too long.
78	Mr. James:	Yeah.
79	Dr. D:	And that's when we say, okay, we can go the next step.
80	Mr. James:	Yeah.
81		Definitely.
82		That's it.

Dr. D (lines 65–68) continues to share the direction of the path with his overall assessment that Mr. James is doing very well. This enables Mr. James to acknowledge the team. 'In the land of dissimilitude I am alone but not isolated'. Recognizing the Others as being part of one's own process of

---

[6]Please refer to Chapter 2 for a description of Heidegger's (1927/1962) *aufsässig (obstinate)* and *aufdringlich (obtrusive)*.

[7]Winnicott's holding function of parent-infant relationship (Winnicott, 1960) transported into the medical environment transforms the encounter into a therapeutic/healing relation.

[8]For safety reasons, in this university hospital, every patient discharged after VAD or transplant surgery is required to live within an hour's-drive radius from the hospital during the first three months postoperatively.

making sense of the land of dissimilitude constitutes a transformation from *selva oscura* to *selva antica*. These Others are not there to tell us things we do not understand, we do not recognize, or we are afraid of. Mr. Montale, in Chapter 1, concludes: *"Geee can I possibly ever come out of this? But the staff, the doctor I met and my wife's strength . . . I came out. I came out of there"*. These others are an integral part of what is becoming familiar, our life.

On the basis of the synchronization of perspectives, Dr. D understands that Mr. James has a sense of the horizon, Dr. D, at line 72 with the two-second-long pause, now finetunes the plan. He provides reliable images of what the path as a whole looks like as it can develop in time (line 74) and space (line 75), how to envision the next step on the path, i.e., to be listed on the active heart transplant waiting list.

Mr. James is not 'just fine' (line 3), he is on a path with Dr. D at his side.

The physical examination in the RelationalAct

The interval history (Fauci, 2008), as a part of the *continuation phase* of the Relational*Act* encounter, is concluded and Dr. D moves into the physical examination part.

83	Dr. D:	Let me listen to you.
84		When are your parents coming in?
85	Mr. James:	Uhh, they should be here in the next 30 to 45 minutes.
86	Dr. D:	Ah, okay, that's good.
87		*Dr. D auscultates Mr. James and conducts the routine hand squeeze, the routine visit continues while patient and Dr. D also resume the conversation.*
88		Squeeze my hands as hard as you can, show me your potential.
89		Great!

The hand squeeze: Dr. D crosses his hands at the elbows and asks Mr. James to squeeze both of his hands as hard as Mr. James can. In all other encounters we have analyzed, the omnipresent hand squeeze is usually introduced by: "Please squeeze my hands as hard as you can. Don't be shy, show me your potential." This is Dr. D's heart test in the land of high-tech modern medicine: a simple cross hand-squeeze.

In CoGen, Dr. D says: "It tells me a lot about the patient's emotional preparedness to live." The function of the hand squeeze is threefold: (1) to assess the patient's neurological competence, i.e., rule out a potential stroke, (2) to test the muscular strength, including a test of frailty, which gives important indications on how an individual will be able to mobilize forces to face and fight through the upcoming health crisis and challenges. It is a very good sign when a patient who squeezes Dr. D's hands says, as Mrs. Dove, a 58-year-old patient, repeatedly did during her convalescence from heart transplantation surgery: "Doctor, I could have done it harder but I didn't want to hurt you." That patient is prepared to fight for life. With the best medicine and the best surgical interventions, if a person cannot continue to fight to be healthy and loses the autopoietic potential (Varela, Maturana, & Uribe, 1974), the energy and desire to live, health professionals are helpless. Dr. D continues: "In whoever dies a spiritual death, physical death will follow". (3) The third function of the hand squeeze is to establish "agency over the healthcare system, which is to be squeezed, to be used in support of the patient, the *person*care": the healthcare system as a *ready-to-hand* tool.

90	Dr. D:	Lasix helped you said this morning right?
91	Mr. James:	Yeah, yeah, yeah, after I wake up,
92		after a couple hours of sleep,
93		I peed out 20 ounces of fluid (2.0 s).
94	Dr. D:	Uh-huh.
95	Mr. James:	[not understandable]
96		And then I had to go again
97		and I put out other 14, 15 ounces.
98	Dr. D:	Uhm uh (3.0 s).
99		Sit up for a moment please.
100		*Dr. D continues conducting the physical examination auscultating the back.*
101	Dr. D:	Take a deep breath.
102	Mr. James:	I can also breathe deeper than I could yesterday too.
103	Dr. D:	Yeah.

With the physical examination, the encounter *continuation phase* concludes. Dr. D feels he has updated all the relevant information with Mr. James: Mr. James' medical well-being, all the relevant interrelated experiences of disease and illness; together they created for Mr. James and Dr. D important steps required to continues to engage in the ever-developing path in healing. It is time to conclude the encounter with the next specific action steps.

Conclusion Phase

104	Dr. D:	So
105		when your parents come you have me beeped,
106		I am around
107		in one of the other rooms.
108	Mr. James:	Okay.
109	Dr. D:	I come and we sit and talk.
110	Mr. James:	Sounds good.
111	Dr. D:	I see you then.
112	Mr. James:	Sounds good.

The *conclusion phase* of the Relational*Act* serves the purpose of guaranteeing that the encounter ends with the synchronized consensual action steps for the path ahead. It is important to reiterate that any consensus reached is not elaborated in the framework of choice but in framework of care (Mackenzie & Stoljar, 2000; Mol, 2008). There will be no moral normatives organizing Dr. D's evaluation of Mr. James' behavior in relation to his adherence to the steps agreed upon today, but it continues to be, as discussed at the beginning of this chapter, an imperative for Dr. D to care.

So what will happen if the next time Dr. D enters Mr. James' room and finds that despite having increased the dose of Lasix (line 90), Mr. James still did not walk or sit, as specified by the regimen for recovery? Dr. D's practice of high-tech modern medicine requires learning to guide integration of treatments, goals and technological advancement *iteratively* into *this specific person's* life. And it is this integration that Dr. D will have to continue to assist with, as we saw in this chapter developing during the meeting on Day 9 of post-BiVAD implantation. Yes, nobody said it was easy.

The Evolution of the Encounter

Two months later, Mr. James has fully recovered from the BiVAD surgery and is scheduled in the afternoon for a visit in the *out*patient VAD clinic at the hospital.

Very early that morning, on the same day of Mr. James' scheduled visit, Dr. D receives a phone call with a heart offer, possibly a good match for Mr. James. The parameters seem okay; the heart is functioning. There is always that small chance, the small chance that upon the physical inspection by the donor team, the heart will turn out not to be of the necessary quality for transplantation. But so far, the parameters seem okay; the heart is functioning.

Hope.

While the donor organ team is called to inspect the heart accepted for Mr. James, Mr. James himself receives the phone call: a donor heart has become available. Mr. James must urgently come to the hospital. As per safety protocol, for the first three months following the mechanical assist device implantation, Mr. James has temporarily relocated along with his family to a place within a one-hour driving distance from the hospital, rather than in his residence much farther away. Upon arrival at the CTICU, preparation for Mr. James' surgery starts. He will not be able to drink or eat for many hours. And now, he and his family wait: a heart, a new heart, no BiVAD, no click, clack, click, clack, going home, finally.

A few hours later, the result: the donor heart is not of the expected quality. The heart is not accepted for Mr. James' transplantation: a dry run.

Mr. James remains in the CTICU (now Day 81 after BiVAD implantation) for what was originally planned to be a routinely scheduled *out*patient clinic appointment. Dr. D enters, prepared to address Mr. James' disappointment; as he knows, it can be devastating for a patient and the family to receive the phone call to come to the hospital for the heart offer and, as in Mr. James' case, wait with high hope; hope, mixed with fear that the surgery could have bad outcomes, hope mixed with guilt that somebody had to die to give the heart and hope that they will soon be celebrating a new life and finally going back home.

But now, a 'dry run'.

Dr. D knows that after the experience of a dry run any person can go into a depression.

Mr. James has already gone through a rough course, as it is the nature of the disease and now he experiences the disappointment of the dry run. Actually, there is more.

When a heart offer is received by the recipient patient's transplantation center, a patient is called as Mr. James was, and he/she needs to decide whether to accept the offer. At this moment, a patient is obtrusively confronted with the reality of his/her own heart as a piece of *obstinate unready-to-hand* equipment (Heidegger, 1927/1962) that is, in this case a heart that is not only malfunctioning but needs to be replaced altogether, a broken tool impeding this person's life. After the evaluation, and recommendation for heart transplantation listing a patient knows that his/her own heart will be replaced sometime in the future. This notion slowly becomes part of the patient's life as he/she and also his/her family becomes more familiar with this understanding. This notion becomes familiar as understanding of a new life, that is, a life where one can walk, run, take showers, swim, go to the opera, make love without bruising the loved one etc.; a way of life. Now, however, with the heart offer call, a patient is confronted with the decision to eliminate some equipment that is not working and substitute it with another. This is what we would do with a hammer whose head has come off; we get a new one. But, in our context of advanced heart failure, it is one's own body, one's own heart. The patient from having a sense about her/his own life must focus on making sense of being of substitutable body parts.

As he prepares to meet Mr. James, Dr. D's 'data' material for this encounter's *preparation phase*, is richer in details, as Dr. D and Mr. James have now known each other for more than two months. Dr. D enters the CTICU room, knowing that Mr. James has already received the 'dry run' news.

1	Dr. D:	Hi young man.
2	Mr. James:	Howdy.
3	Dr. D:	He:y (1.0 s)
4		what a beautiful view of the whole man.
5		(5.2 s)
6	Mr. James:	Glad that I'm awake.
7	Dr. D:	(1.4) How are you?
8		(1.0 s)
9	Mr. James:	Good. (1.8 s)

A 'beautiful view of the whole man' (line 4) is the first thing Dr. D tells Mr. James. What a strange thing to say, yet Dr. D is conveying something positive; his tone of voice, as we hear it in the recordings also conveys something positive. While Mr. James could have the perspective 'now something went seriously wrong', a perspective of a great disappointment, Dr. D wants to let him know that this is part of a big-picture plan within which everything looks overall very good. To do so, Dr. D proposes a positive view of Mr. James that does not minimize the disappointment; there is no '*yes* you are disappointed, *but* think about the big picture', no yes-*but* type of message, presupposing that one is not thinking in the right way about one's own experience, rather, Dr. D has only a positive message for Mr. James to hear. This is important because the '*but* think about the big picture' part is not Mr. James' elaborated perspective. It is the medical perspective of a course of the disease and its therapeutic options that presupposes possibilities of dry runs or other complications in the larger perspective of long-term survival.

In the *initiation phase* of this encounter, there is not the open question 'how is life,' as in other encounters. In those encounters it is necessary to open a space in which the patient selects the first topic in the medical conversation; the patient's answer together with the other elements discussed above constitute a critical diagnostic assembled at the person level. In this encounter with Mr. James however, the pressing need is to immediately address the possible issue of disappointment, by confronting reality and opening up the path for hope.

Five seconds of silence (line 5) are left for Mr. James, who does not elaborate beyond line 6. If we take Mr. James' loquacious style of conversation in Chapter 2 (on Day 10 postoperatively, e.g., *initiation phase* lines 1–10) as representative of his style in the encounters with Dr. D, we could, with Dr. D, interpret the 5.2 seconds of silence in the current *initiation phase* as a message that Mr. James is in the land of dissimilitude. How to proceed into the *continuation phase*?

10	Dr. D:	So (2.2 s)
11		the reason obviously (0.8 s)
12		before you even had your clinical appointment this afternoon
13		when we were going to meet
14		and you came a little earlier was
15		as you know that the heart offer,
16		a heart became available.
17	Mr. James:	Hmm hmm.
18	Dr. D:	(1.2 s) Well, everything looked good
19		until the organ turned out to be not of sufficient good quality.
20		(1.4 s)
21		So that's why we had to decline this one.
22		(1.3 s)
23		This tells us
24		things are coming up
25		and it could be (1 s)
26		coming up
27		any moment.
28	Mr. James:	Okay
29	Dr. D:	You know.

As Mr. James, in the land of dissimilitude, listens to Dr. D without any talk overlap or interruption, he needs to know that Dr. D can recognize him in the land of dissimilitude and see the path unfolding.

In the *preparation* and *initiation phases* of this encounter, the expected/observed comparison serves to prepare Dr. D to deliver, upfront and early in the encounter, three statements in one coherent piece: (1) there was a heart offer (line 15), (2) it was not good enough for you (lines 19–21) and (3) there will soon be another offer that is going to be good for you. To address the disappointment and give hope, Dr. D gives these messages in this order, before anything else happens in the encounter. As he reports in CoGen, Dr. D concludes the introduction statement with a sense of 'Okay this did not work. You can be sure we will only take the best for you and there are things coming up, that is, the fact that this heart was offered to you gives us confidence that there will be other offers'. In this situation Dr. D has a strong sense to get the three messages across right away because for Mr. James, as it would be for any patient, the 'dry run' can be devastating; a loss of hope that can turn agency, the potential to face and fight through the possible upcoming health crisis, into disillusionment.

30	Dr. D:	Bu::t (1.2 s)
31		I hope it was not too disappointing to you.
32		(1 s) How
33		how did you experience it when you received the call.
34		You received the call when you texted me.
35		You texted me right after.
36	Mr. James:	Yeah.
37	Dr. D:	Because I was the one who took the organ offer.
38	Mr. James:	Oh, okay.
39		Hmm (1.6 s)
40		I don't know.
41		It was kind of weird.
42		Hmm (2.6 s)
43		u(hh) u(hh) (laughter)
44		I was kind of expected to be at VAD clinic (outpatient visit)
45		[or]
46	Nurse:	[Hi]

Note that on line 30, as on line 3 for 'He::y', we use the notation '::' to indicate a stretched sound of the vowel 'u', as this notation helps in indicating that the sound of the word is longer and less definitive. Dr. D moves to ask Mr. James to share his experience with the dry run. It is a direct question and as we will discuss in Chapter 4, less expert doctors not addressing the disappointment immediately, or worse, not addressing it at all, may leave the patient and the family having to reconstitute a sense for a path by themselves, that is, in the land of dissimilitude where they are not recognized and helped.

At line 45, a nurse enters to attend to the BiVAD and the conversation now alternates between the experience of life with a BiVAD and how knowledgeable and proficient Mr. James and his family have become, managing the BiVAD, changing the battery, dealing with the BiVAD alarms, etc., while the experience of the 'dry run' is woven into the conversation by Dr. D. Dr. D asks and discusses questions emerging from this specific encounter relevant to Mr. James' and his family's experiences. Learning to care in action: the dry run, the BiVAD, these experiences as Mr. James' father drives as fast as he safely can to get to the hospital, the charging of the battery, are actions that Mr. James and his parents do and do *together*. It is in doing or conceiving of one doing things that things, gestures, actions enter our relational world and become familiar (Heidegger, 1927/1962). The dry run has to be integrated in the life of Mr. James and his family in order not to overshadow all their lives.

Two weeks later (Day 99 after BiVAD implantation), after having reviewed the medical situation with the CTICU team, Dr. D is preparing to enter Mr. James' room. Dr. D is excited: the night before, Mr. James underwent heart transplantation. As the pictures Mr. James asked the surgeon to take during his transplantation surgery show (Figures 3.1 and 3.2), Mr. James' own heart and the two assist pumps were removed from his body by the heart surgeon and a new heart from another person was sewn in. While all this was going on, Mr. James was intubated and was on the breathing machine as well as on the heart and lung machine that temporarily replaced his lung and heart functions during the transplantation surgery. Now, on the morning after the surgery, the breathing machine has already been removed and Mr. James is extubated and talking. A very fast recovery; Mr. James' voice is very hoarse because of the inflammation associated with intubation. Dr. D knows that getting extubated is a critical moment (see Chapter 4), and it went well.

No breathing machine, no heart and lung machine, and no BiVAD. Mr. James has a new heart. Dr. D is excited entering the room and expects

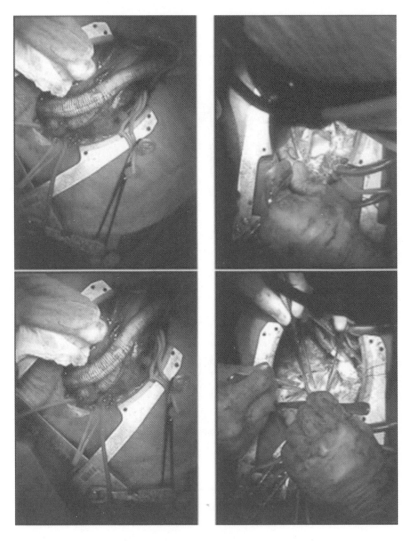

Figure 3.1: Mr. James undergoing heart transplantation: BiVAD-explantation. The rippled tubes (cannulae) are the inflow and outflow BiVAD graft connecting the pump to heart, and big vessels: aorta LVAD and pulmonary artery RVAD.

(*preparation phase*) Mr. James and his family to be celebrating. Mr. James' father and a social worker on-call are with Mr. James in the room.

1	Dr. D:	So where is the young man?
2		What a beautiful moment!
3	Mr. James:	Yes!

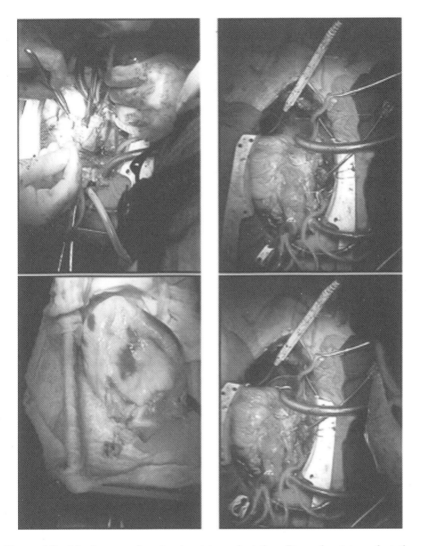

Figure 3.2: Mr. James undergoing heart transplantation: Donor heart transplantation (details see text).

4	Dr. D:	Young man.
5		Hi.
6	Social Worker:	Hi.
7	Dr. D:	Good morning sir (playfully bows).
8		Welcome to the new life!
9	Mr. James:	Thank you!
10		[Date removed] is my new birthday.

11	Social Worker:	That's it.
12	Dr. D:	You are wonderful.
13		To see you like this
14		the morning after the transplant
15		exhaling on your own.
16	Mr. James:	Yes.
17	Dr. D:	In-cre-di-ble.
18		Congratulations!
19	Mr. James:	Thank you.
20	Dr. D:	And the whole team feels like that.
21		Hugs from everyone.
22		So any thoughts?
23	Mr. James:	Any thoughts,
24		I would like to be able to drink
25		a whole big gallon of ice water right now.
26		That'd be just the most wonderful thing.
27	Dr. D:	Wow.
28	Social Worker:	It's not gonna happen, eh?
29	Dr. D:	Eh n:o.
30	Mr. James:	I kno::w.
31	Dr. D:	Isn't it beautiful!
32		Looks like a same day procedure.
33	Mr. James:	(Laughing) Marines core manifesting itself.
34		(3 s)
35	Dr. D:	Having said that, during the
36		next 99 years you will have this or that going on
37		a bit rejections, a bit infections, b[it of] this and that.
38	Mr. James:	[Yeah]
39	Dr. D:	So (1 s)
40		that is not a problem just
41	Mr. James:	just life now.
42	Dr. D:	Just,
43	Dr. D:	but now we can start on [Mr. James' home town-removed] planning
44	Mr. James:	Yes!

In the first encounter right after heart transplantation, a patient can be either very excited or not excited. If the patient is not excited which Dr. D finds out during the *initiation phase* — for example because the pain is making the person feel as if the body is made of broken parts, *obtrusive* — then the goal will be to move the patient towards the perspective of a new life with the new heart. Yes, it is a new life because a person with the advanced heart disease has been severely limited in every daily experience, from walking to eating, when food has lost the taste it had before, taking a shower, standing in front of a mirror and shaving can become an ordeal; and as in Mr. James' case, accepting to live with a machine 'weirded him out'. Yes, a new life, to rc-lcarn to live.

If, as it happens, a patient is overly euphoric and excited, then the goal in the *continuation phase* is to integrate, in this very encounter moment, the long-term perspective and the anticipated challenges of living with high doses of immunosuppression medications, the high chances of infection and the need to constantly monitor oneself for rejection and organ dysfunction.

We report this encounter here, as we want to illustrate how *continuation phases* can change dynamics in response to the *initiation phase*. In this *continuation phase*, after sharing the excitement about the heart transplantation, Dr. D wants to use the energy of the excitement for the moment, to create a long-term perspective for Mr. James, the life with the new heart, the long-term post-transplantation course (line 36). As discussed in the CoGen session, Dr. D's intention is to make Mr. James feel that, although there will be rejection, infection, and organ dysfunction episodes, these will not reduce 'the overall beautiful long-term perspective'. Note that on line 35 Dr. D introduces the "bumpiness" without using terms such as "but" or "however" which could denote a contrast to the "normal" course. As he describes in CoGen: "So, the 100-year perspective image is powerful for the patient because I don't want this personal moment of joy to be translated into utopia: it is in this moment of euphoria that one can incorporate the idea of little bumpiness as a component, an integral part of the overall long-term perspective." The goal is to integrate scientific technological advancement into Mr. James' *personal* life.

CHAPTER 4
PROTECTING THE *DYAD*
IN PRACTICE

Ms. Loy is 43. She has been very active in building her career as an architect. Her heart failure syndrome deteriorated until she was so sick that she had to urgently be transferred to the hospital where Dr. D works. There, Ms. Loy is evaluated for heart transplantation and listed on the high emergency category UNOS 1A heart transplantation waiting list. She remains in the CCU until transplantation. Part of the treatment is a continuous infusion of two heart-strengthening medications whose effects are continuously monitored through measurements of blood flow and heart pressures through a right heart catheter. The catheter, made of plastic, needs to be changed every ten days to prevent blood stream infection. Two nights before encountering Dr. D, a compatible donor heart became available and preparation for her heart transplantation surgery began, with Ms. Loy fasting for some hours before surgery. But it was a dry run; Ms. Loy was not transplanted. Dr. D who starts attending today, rounds with another cardiologist whom he is mentoring, Dr. Arbeet. The two doctors had briefly introduced themselves to Ms. Loy and her parents the day before, announcing that they would be on rounds for the next 14 consecutive days. Ms. Loy's parents are in the hospital room with her when Dr. Arbeet and Dr. D enter:

Day 1

1	Dr. Arbeet:	Hello Ms. Loy.
2		How are you doing?
3		Oh you got the fish huh?
4		(2 s)

For the following half minute the conversation moves from 'the traveling fish' — a goldfish the nurses in the CCU offer to put in a patient's room if s/he so desires — to a group of medical students who have been shadowing the cardiologists during rounds.

A comparison with the *initiation phase* examples we discussed in Chapter 3 immediately brings attention to a question/assertion on line 3 right after the opening question on line 2. There is no silence, no space for Ms. Loy or her parents to answer the question on line 2. With no silence after line 2, line 3 closes the opportunity at the opening.

At line 21 with a clear signal 'So...', Dr. Arbeet concludes the talk about the fish and medical students. Line 21 changes the conversation to a problem presentation framework, a rapid move also observed in general practice (Heritage & Maynard, 2006). Dr. Arbeet asks a question regarding the procedure of changing the right heart catheter the day before this encounter. Ms. Loy, still experiencing pain, has been prescribed pain medication (Vicodin):

21	Dr. Arbeet:	So how are you feeling?
22	Ms. Loy:	Um-hm (1.0s)
23		I'm on Vicodin but
24		so didn't sleep very well last night.
25		Besides that (1.0s)
26	Dr. Arbeet:	So, the site of insertions?
27	Ms. Loy:	The site and
28		um-hm (1.0s)
29		I think when he went in
30		I could feel it against my throat
31		which is why I think my voice is like this.
32		This has been poking.
33		Because like when you did it on this side,
34		I had a pain in my shoulder blade
35		from where I think it made a corner or something
36		and I think that's what this is
37		it made a corner.
38	Dr. D:	Yeah.
39	Dr. Arbeet:	Yes, but the pain is controlled with the Vicodin?
40	Ms. Loy:	Oh yea.
41	Dr. Arbeet:	All right, uhh.
42	Ms. Loy:	Hhh.hhh.hhh.hhhh (*laughter*).
43	Dr. Arbeet:	Any other issues? Any other problems?
44	Ms. Loy:	Hmmm, [no]
45	Dr. Arbeet:	[So] from our perspective
46		there's not much to report to you.
47	Ms. Loy:	[Okay]
48	Dr. Arbeet:	[Uhhh] everything is pretty stable
49		and we're waiting for the phone call
50		so we can get the heart.

51	Mother:	Okay. The good one. The perfect one.
52	Dr. Arbeet:	Yah.
53		Okay then.

One and half minutes into the encounter, Dr. Arbeet is concluding and just about ready to exit the room (line 53). Dr. D intervenes (line 54); Ms. Loy just went through a dry run and the experience needs to be discussed. As an emotionally traumatic event, the attending cardiologists need to be sure that Ms. Loy, as well as her parents, are putting the dry run in a perspective where healing is on the horizon:

54	Dr. D:	Yeah and now
55		you know already what it means to go through a dry run (1.5 s)
56		and
57		did you know how that feels
58		you know going through this then ...
59	Mother:	I did anesthesia so I felt pretty good.
60	Dr. D:	Yeah I know.
61	Father:	Yeah, well we got a dry run too so
62	Dr. D:	Yes that's why I'm asking
63		from your perspective (parents)
64		but also from yours, right? (Ms. Loy)
65	Father:	Yes.
66	Dr. D:	You get ready and then ...
67	Father:	Yes.
68	Ms. Loy:	That's what I told him (father)
69		you know,
70		it's the emotional part you know of the whole thing,
71	Dr. D:	Um-hm.
72	Ms. Loy:	especially since it happened so fast.
73	Dr. D:	Um-hm. Yeah.

Dr. D is engaging Ms. Loy and her parents at the same time (lines 54–58). Ms. Loy is not talking. As Ms. Loy's mother is also a doctor and anesthesiologist, Dr. D (lines 57–58) addresses her directly, as he wants to be sure that she, also in her role of physician, is in agreement on the medical level. If this does not happen, the conversation between Ms Loy's mother (anesthesiologist) and doctor (cardiologist) has the potential to take two directions that would not benefit the patient: it could become rather esoteric, excluding all others, the patient and other family members, from the conversation and maintaining it exclusively on the technical medical level. It could also become antagonistic, with the two physicians competing for the appreciation of competency by daughter/patient. If either of these directions is taken in the conversation, the patient has little, if no, chance to voice her perspective and needs. The conversation in this form cannot integrate the biomedical science into the person level of the 'here and now' needs of the patient.

As Dr. Arbeet did not complete this encounter task, Dr. D re-engages Ms. Loy and her parents in the conversation (lines 63–64) to create a safe space, an explicit invitation to patient and her parents to feel comfortable to discuss and share their experience with the dry run. Five minutes later in the encounter, Ms. Loy will ask if Dr. D will be in the operating room during her transplantation surgery. From Dr. D's perspective, this question indicates that Ms. Loy feels comfortable with him and trusts him.

154	Ms. Loy:	So will you be in the actual surgery?

How did we get to the point of the question (line 154) signaling that the patient trusts the doctor?

90	Mother:	You know the anesthesiologist came out to the waiting room
91		I'm like something has happened
92		either something bad or something b[:ad]
93	Dr. D:	[Ooo]h
94	Mother:	you know
95	Dr. D:	yeah.
96		So this is ehh among bad things,
97		the best that could happen.
98	Ms. Loy:	Yeah.
99	Father:	Yeah.
100	Mother:	Yeah.
101	Father:	Well
102		and like she says, (0.9)
103		it's not all that bad to find out.
104	Dr. D:	No,
105		exactly right.
106	Ms. Loy:	Before, while it was well outside my body
107		not inside my body.
108	Dr. D:	Um-hm
109		um-hm
110		um-hm
111		um-hm.

The experience of going for a dry run is a difficult one for everyone, Ms. Loy and her parents. It entails preparation to exchange one's own heart for somebody else's heart, a donor heart which is a difficult passage in a patient's life and subsequently coping with the disappointment of not being able to make the critical transition into the next phase of one's own life. As we also discussed in Chapter 3 when Mr. James had a dry run, in this moment a patient is *obtrusively* confronted with the reality of his own heart as *unready-to-hand* equipment (Heidegger, 1927/1962), a heart as a broken tool to be replaced as it is impeding life. As this notion is transformed slowly into something that is more familiar to the patient and her family as a potential for a new life, when the heart offer call is received, the patients and often the family are confronted with the decision to eliminate the 'equipment' (the patient's own heart) that is not working and substituting it with another in one's own body. In this experience, Ms. Loy as well as her parents must be supported in moving from focusing on making sense of being composed of substitutable broken body parts to having a sense about her own life, as Dr. D does on lines 114–119 below.

The 'dry run' has been upgraded to 'goldfish status' (line 3)! The subject is back to what was supposed to be discussed at the beginning of the encounter. Here, as we saw him doing in Chapter 3, transforming into a 'big thing' what Mr. James called 'weird' (in reference to being implanted with a BiVAD), Dr. D does also a transformation on lines 96–97, of 'bad' into 'best that can happen', which is followed by the agreement statements of Ms. Loy and her parents. The conversation continues with Dr. D leaving space for Ms. Loy and her parents to talk (lines 90–111).

112	Mother:	For some reason I thought if all the tests went all right
113		it couldn't.
114	Dr. D:	I mean
115		the situation is by the nature of organ transplantation
116		such that while you're being prepared
117		a second team in parallel, same time
118		in the donor hospital is preparing the donor organ
119		and until you guys meet and everything is one
120		you know
121		things can happen at any stage in the process.
122	Ms. Loy:	Is there a specific general hospital or are there specific ones [or]
123	Dr. D:	[No]
124	Ms. Loy:	just any hospital?
125	Dr. D:	any hospital and you know the United States is divided in
126		like umm to make [possible] the work
127		of the United Network for Organ Sharing
128		which is based on the organ transplantation law of 1986
129		a kind of comprehensive national eh law eh in 60 different organ

130		procurement organization areas.
131		And ours here in [region's name]
132		the organ procurement organization [name],
133		is the largest one,
134		you know if you have 60 of these in 300 million,
135		on average you have 5 million inhabitants per organization and
136		we have in our region 20 million,
137	Ms. Loy:	Wow.
138	Dr. D:	and it's about umm 200 or so hospitals you know,
139	Ms. Loy:	Okay.
140	Dr. D:	you know
141		that could call and say you know, we have a situation here and so.
142	Ms. Loy:	So there's no time in having the transport.
143	Dr. D:	No and so
144		that's why you know while there's a national waiting list
145		if we get information
146	Ms. Loy:	Yea, that's in a whole different, yes.
147	Dr. D:	and it all goes in a very algorithm-based way uhm
148		there's at the same time a continuous update
149		in the donor hospital on how things are
150		and until it's done, it's not done, so, you know?
151	Ms. Loy:	Hhh.hhh.hhh.hhhh.
152	Dr. D:	That's the overall idea.
153	Mother:	That sounds good.
154	Ms. Loy:	So will you be in the actual surgery?

Once again, it is Ms. Loy's mother steering the conversation (line 112) into an area that she perceives might be of importance for her daughter, the patient: the logistics of heart transplantation in the U.S. While an explanation of the process had been provided to Ms. Loy and her parents earlier, in preparation for Ms. Loy's placement on the waiting list, going over the situation again in this moment after Ms. Loy's experience of the dry run and pointing out that dry runs are part of the routine of heart transplantation, is an important, trust-creating step: Ms. Loy asks if Dr. D will be present during her heart transplantation surgery (line 154). Note that Dr. D takes the suggestion from Ms. Loy's mother (line 112) as a good starting point to talk with Ms. Loy, whom he addresses directly. This is important because Dr. D recognizes that the input from Ms. Loy's family, in this case Ms. Loy's mother, is important, as she knows her daughter better than Dr. D does. Starting from this input, Dr. D continues to address Ms. Loy directly, maintaining the dyad between doctor and patient as the privileged relationship. Dr. D's explanation has a specific structure: it is a story; it has a space in which the process develops, a time required for the process to develop, and the dependence on the interconnectivity of the participants. The explanation is then always given in the context where it is part of the patient's and family's experience and with appropriate level of details. In this specific moment, in this patient's and family's experience, the function of this explanation is to make the patient and family comfortable in knowing that the chance of having the next donor offer soon is real (lines 125–138). We call this key element the *explanation* aspect of the encounter.

After the dry run has been integrated as a proper subject in the medical conversation, Dr. D feels that the encounter's *conclusion phase* may proceed and that the patient is well prepared for what will be coming up.

The next day, Dr. Arbeet provides more space for Ms. Loy to answer his question about how she is doing. A little more space, a small step into the right direction immediately followed by a problem presentation question. Nobody said it was easy! No problem to present:

Day 2

1	Dr. Arbeet:	Hello, how are you?
2	Dr. D:	Hello.
3	Mother:	How are you doing?
4	Ms. Loy:	Hello.
5	Dr. Arbeet:	So, how are you doing?
6	Ms. Loy:	Good.
7	Dr. Arbeet:	Any problems overnight?

Dr. Arbeet, then trying to close the encounter after less than a minute (line 19 below), is called back by Ms. Loy's signal that the encounter is not over (line 24).

Ms. Loy's laughter at line 21, as soon as Dr. Arbeet makes the closing statement at line 20, also signals a discrepancy between Dr. Arbeet's understanding that all is well and that he can leave and Ms. Loy's need for more communication. Studies in conversation analysis have shown that patients in medical conversation can signal, with laughter, that the conversation at hand is delicate and often use it to remedy an interactional problem (Haakana, 2001). As this laughter neither follows a joke nor is part of a joyful moment within which it would be an integral part of the conversation, we interpret it as a remedy to an interactional problem.

Day 2

19	Dr. Arbeet	Okay.
20		Well we don't have much news for you.
21	Ms. Loy:	Hhh.hhh.hhh.hhhh (laugher)
22	Dr. Arbeet:	We just wanted to stop by and say hello
23		and see if there's anything we can do for you.
24	Ms. Loy:	I'm just waiting
25		and you know I know this is part of it.
26		It's all a part of it.
27	Dr. Arbeet:	Yea.
28	Ms. Loy:	Hhh.hhh.hhh.hhhh
29	Dr. Arbeet:	Yea.
30	Dr. D:	There will be news coming up (1.5 s).
31		But we don't yet know exactly when.
32	Ms. Loy	Yes.
33		(1.4 s)

After a second laughter by Ms. Loy (line 28) and Dr. D's statement (lines 30–31), Dr. Arbeet, now listening with more attention, abandons his move to close the encounter. Dr. D, in response to Ms. Loy's laughter, indicates that he knows she is worried about the uncertainty of the time point of receiving a donor heart offer (line 30) and assures her that heart transplantation will happen.

Dr. Arbeet, attuning to Dr. D signaling that the encounter is not over, proceeds to continue it (line 34) with questions regarding Ms. Loy's physical well-being.

34	Dr. Arbeet:	And you are getting up and walking around and
35	Ms. Loy:	I, I got up uhm.
36		The other day I walked for
37		like an hour-and-a-half around
38		when they changed when I was free.
39	Dr. D:	Yeah.
40	Ms. Loy:	And like this morning I got up
41		and did some exercises and some stretching
42		I lifted my water bottle.
43	Dr. Arbeet:	And any bowel movements?
44	Ms. Loy:	Had one today.
45	Dr. Arbeet:	Yeah.
46	Ms. Loy:	Hhh.hhh.hhh.hhhh (laughs)
47	Dr. Arbeet:	Okay,
48		yeah excellent.
49	Ms. Loy:	I think I'm okay.

50	Dr. Arbeet:	Alright cool,
51		we will just keep our fingers crossed.
52	Ms. Loy:	Yeah just before everything starts moving again I know I'll be.

As we said, it is not easy. Dr. Arbeet continues by asking about Ms. Loy's bowel movements, part of what, in CoGen, the doctors called 'the checklist' learned in medical school. This is of particular relevance in Ms. Loy's current situation, because there is no medical reason for a cardiologist to revert to questions that an intern asks and, in intensive care units, the nurses monitor continually. In contrast, it could be the topic of the medical encounter after an event such as a surgery. As a reaction to the medication administered during surgery, e.g., pain control medication, it may be difficult for a patient to have bowel movements causing potentially serious complications for the patient. But this is not the case here and Ms. Loy is still not done talking to the doctors. After Dr. Arbeet tries to close the encounter for the second time, she continues talking (line 52).

Dr. D intervenes, asking both Ms. Loy and her mother if they have any questions; no they do not; Dr. D then asks where Ms. Loy's parents are staying while their daughter is in the hospital waiting for transplantation. Dr. Arbeet is becoming attuned to Dr. D's cues and picks up on them during this part of the encounter — *continuation phase*. He follows up by asking where Ms. Loy's parents' home is located and where Ms. Loy lives. The conversation now comes to an important point as Dr. Arbeet shares with Ms. Loy that he visited the town in which Ms. Loy lives. Ms. Loy learns that Dr. Arbeet had stayed as a guest in the hotel she had designed. Ms. Loy tells him that it was the last work she did before being admitted to the hospital. Dr. Arbeet acknowledges her professional work and specifically underscores the beauty of the hotel that the patient had designed. This is, as we have discussed, a very important step as it relates to *this patient's life*. Dr. Arbeet continues:

116	Dr. Arbeet:	Yea.
117		But I heard that the numbers were going down
118		and now they're [starting]
119	Ms. Loy:	[They're starting] to show a profit.
120	Dr. Arbeet:	Really?
121	Ms. Loy:	Last quarter.
122	Dr. Arbeet:	Oh wow.

Here, Dr. Arbeet does not maintain the *dyadic* coherence that he initially created.

The Function of the Dyad

An important function of the dyad at this point in the medical encounter is to support the patient's recovery, helping Ms. Loy to *integrate* her experience in advanced heart failure with her future heart transplantation and her societal/professional life post-transplantation. Dr. Arbeet, as shown above, enters into a framework that breaks the function of the dyad and fragments Ms. Loy's experience into *separated* bits: illness, work, disease. There is no need to talk about the shares or the managerial success of the hotel team because it is not part of Ms. Loy's accomplishment. She designed it. As the encounter proceeds, Dr. Arbeet is not able to integrate them.

So how to change this? In CoGen session, the physicians recounted finding themselves in similar common situations and discussed the possible opening of the situation toward integration in Ms. Loy's life of her experience with advanced heart failure, and the changes a physician can make in relating to a patient. One possibility discussed in CoGen was to help Ms. Loy recall the positive impact of her work on others. In this specific example, the physician had personally enjoyed the product of her work (the hotel) and the discussion on this should have stopped after thanking Ms. Loy for her work, as she thanked the doctors for their work. By doing so, a clear recognition of the person's professional identity is offered. The next step is to return this retrieved professional image/identity into the medical encounter, providing a sense of the path that is relevant to this patient, Ms. Loy, who, in this moment, is waiting in the hospital for heart transplantation, away from her work, her house, her life and with a dry run experience a couple days earlier. This step of returning the recalled image/identity into the medical encounter has the function of maintaining and protecting the dyad in order to optimally care for Ms. Loy. For example, Dr. Arbeet could have asked the following question: 'How is your perspective after recovering from heart transplantation, are you going to continue with your beautiful work in the same city/same company?' The answer to this question would provide the physician with an important basis for an integrated plan for the first three months after transplantation, when Ms. Loy, as the other patients, will need to live near the hospital, and the transition to life in the long term, post-transplantation. This move would provide a visualization of the steps on the path to Ms. Loy's full recovery in a life that she recognizes as hers, completely integrated within Ms. Loy's societal/professional context.

Ten days later, that is, after four weeks of waiting in the intensive care unit, Ms. Loy is successfully transplanted. She wakes up after heart transplantation surgery and is extubated within 24 hours.

Her mother is with her in the CTICU room. Dr. D is still attending and rounds with Dr. Arbeet.

Before entering the room, the two cardiologists have been updating the medical situation with the other advanced heart failure and critical care unit team members. They all agree, Ms. Loy is doing well overall so early postoperatively. She is already extubated (breathing on her own without the breathing machine), which allows her to talk again. Yet, there is some concern over an evolving urgency from the suspected presence of fluid in the pericardial sac that envelops the heart. This condition could impede the filling of the newly transplanted heart with blood (pericardial tamponade) and is potentially a life-threatening situation, that is, at any moment it could lead to the patient coding and requiring resuscitation. Dr. D and Dr. Arbeet order an urgent heart ultrasound (transthoracic echocardiogram) to rule out pericardial tamponade.

Following this *preparation phase* of the encounter, Dr. D and Dr. Arbeet knock at Ms. Loy's door and enter. The encounter's *initiation phase* is starting:

1	Dr. D:	Young lady,
2		congratulations!
3	Ms. Loy:	Thank you.
4		I was just giving bedside manner
5	Dr. Arbeet:	(Dr. Arbeet enters here) Helloo.
6	Mother:	Yes she's been giving bedside manner
7	Ms. Loy:	instructions.
8	Dr. D:	Wonderful.
9	Dr. Arbeet:	You [look]
10	Ms. Loy:	[Eve]n just now.
11	Mother:	Yeah.
12	Dr. Arbeet:	You look good.

Both Dr. D and Dr. Arbeet are relieved (line 12) to see that Ms. Loy is in good shape. She does not look weak and/or feel dizzy, as she could be if the pericardial tamponade were developing. Yet, for Dr. D there is still a discrepancy in the expected/observed comparison. Ms. Loy has just woken up from the long-awaited heart transplantation surgery with a very positive outcome, but the first thing Ms. Loy, followed by her mother, says to the doctors is "I was just giving bedside manner." Noticing this, Dr. D says:

19	Dr. D:	Yea you are so right.
20		And so I think
21		we should all notice that you are beautifully smiling at us.

After listening and acknowledging what Ms. Loy and her mother say (omitted lines 13–18), Dr. D, rather than trying to move the conversation immediately (line 19), transitions the encounter's *initiation phase* to the *continuation phase* (line 20) returning the focus to the important event of heart transplantation in Ms. Loy's life.

When one day after transplantation, there is no crowd of health professionals standing around the patient, when the patient is extubated, and when the patient talks, then Dr. D, as any other doctor would, expects to say: "This is wonderful! Congratulations on your new heart!" The expectation, as we discussed in Chapter 3, is of a celebration. Dr. D expects that the patient would say something like: "Thank you doc! I made it!!!" or might say, with a big smile in her/his eyes, "Yes! We did it!" So, when the physicians hear Ms. Loy saying: "I was just giving bedside manner instructions", (line 4), they think something is wrong; as Dr. D reflects in CoGen: "there is something negative in the situation, I feel that I need to acknowledge it but not by answering directly to it; knowing that the patient is *not* happy and cannot concentrate on this magnificent outcome. When I heard the patient answering this, I felt disappointment; in a fundamental moment of the patient's life where a drastic transformation has happened, from her own diseased heart, through the hours during surgery with no heart in the body, to a new life with a donor heart now beating in the body to keep the patient alive, a patient who now can live her life out of the hospital, at home, at work, with friends and family, the important transformation that nobody really understands emotionally, has been missed." As we have been discussing in previous chapters, this is a difficult transition as the capacity to understand one's own body as *obtrusive* with its broken parts to be substituted (*unreadiness-to-hand*), needs to be transformed into living a life that is one's own. A transformation from body parts to a *person*, being-in-the-world.

A Transformation for the Doctor to Maintain the *Dyad*

On the part of the doctor, it also requires a transformation. Hearing negative statements such as these can give the doctor the sense that the patient does not appreciate the gift they have received from the heart donor, the work of the doctors and nurses, the support of family and also the recognition of the patient's own hard-fought battle and struggles of going through transplantation. A doctor might react by distancing her/himself from the patient and the latter's life's transformation. This sentiment at times can translate also into seeking refuge in the classical asymmetrical power relationship, in which, often involuntarily, the doctor "puts the patient in his place". This kind of reaction neither helps the patient elaborate on her/his own life, nor the doctor's sense of her/his own work. In order to resolve this situation, the doctor needs to say: there is something wrong with my patient and the patient needs help. And then, how to proceed?

The basis for re-synchronization, during the *continuation phase* of this encounter is the understanding on the part of the doctor of her/his role as doctor in encountering the patient. As discussed before, it is not restricted to the knowledge of medical biology and the mere translation of that knowledge into terms that are accessible to non-medical folks. It is much more.

Dr. D's understanding of being a doctor is that of a healthcare professional supporting the patient on his/her journey from the land of dissimilitude into self-determined life, accepting and incorporating the major changes of the body, in this person's life. To this end, independent of whatever negative statements have been made, Dr. D needs to help the patient focus on the situation of having received a heart, of having gone through a major transformation in his/her life.

In response to Ms. Loy's statement "I was giving bedside manners instructions", Dr. D's response, "Wonderful", is a transformation for Dr. D to continue to care for Ms. Loy. This is an important transformation; different from the one we described in Chapters 2 and 3 in the dialogue with Mr. James. The transformation operated with Mr. James had the function of creating a space and a path in which Mr. James could recover from the land of dissimilitude. Here, the transformation is for Dr. D's *selva oscura*. Dr. D needs to transform what he perceives to be a negative statement with the potential, as said above, to make him detach himself from the caring role which would break down his understanding of what being a doctor means to him. Dr. D needs to transform the negative statement with its destructive potential into a space where he can continue to support the *dyadic* connection with Ms. Loy. He operates his own transformation: 1) It is "wonderful" that Ms. Loy can talk, i.e., she is extubated, so soon after heart transplantation and 2) it is "wonderful" that bedside manners are the highest priority for her in that moment, i.e., there is clearly no immediate physical or emotional pain requiring more urgent attention.

In the transition to the *continuation phase*, Dr. D does three things: First, he shares his feedback about the patient's status in a personal way ("First of all, I think we should all notice that you are beautifully smiling at us", line 21). This allows the patient, her mother but also the entire team ("we should all notice") to focus on appreciating the patient's smile at the team, to appreciate the patient as a person, acknowledge her personhood with all personhood-associated properties such as communicating emotions as a starting point and framework of the encounter. This starting point also communicates to the patient that the team is grateful for and values the great outcome.

Second, with the Relational*Act* framework established for patient, for mother, for Dr. D, and for everyone else in the room, Dr. D then proceeds with a suggestion to probe into a more spiritual framing of the situation, implicit in the symbolism of the heart transplantation date on the day of Christmas. This stems from Dr. D's experience with other patients who underwent heart transplantation on symbolic days such as Easter Sunday, and their associations with that symbolism ("And obviously this is December 25th". In other words, "it's very symbolic isn't it?"). However, Ms. Loy does not feel like exploring that symbolism's meaning for her situation in that moment ("Actually the 24th is more for us").

Third, therefore, Dr. D decides to explore another potentially emotionally important aspect of the patient's situation ("... So how was this for you ... I wanna know when you received the information, what the first response was after you had the two dry runs"). Dr. D asks Ms. Loy to recall the previous experience of two dry runs as an integral part of her entire experience in advanced heart failure, as it may be very important for the patient to explore it. This could help her share the potentially traumatic experiences of two heart transplantation offers during the last two weeks that both turned out to be dry runs as the donor organs were not of sufficient quality. Dr. D suspects that the negativity in the initiation phase contained the following meaning: 'I need to have a safe space in which I feel I am being taken seriously as a person because I went through a traumatic experience which I am having a hard time incorporating into my present identity'. This subject then takes the continuation phase through the exploration of the emotional burden experienced during the two dry runs, allowing Ms. Loy to conclude a few minutes later: "I am very pleased with all staff members". As we discussed in Chapter 3, a positive attitude and the energy at the moment of celebration after transplantation form an important part of an emotional framework within which the patient has to learn to incorporate the long-term perspective for life with the new heart. One where there will be instances of complications such as rejection, infection, and organ dysfunction episodes that need to be addressed after the transplantation as they are part of the long-term perspective.

As part of the entire encounter, it is important for Dr. D to try to comprehend the magnitude of what has happened in the life of the patient: How broad is the scope of aspects that must be bridged and how far apart are the ends to connect in this vignette? Forty years after heart transplantation was introduced — still in awe of the wonders of high-tech modern medicine — we are now more mindful of the ontology of being 'thrown into the situation' in an existentialist philosophical sense (Heidegger, 1927/1962). As we discuss throughout the book, the personhood experience in the land of dissimilitude and the high-tech modern medicine experience of body and disease in interaction with technological advancement of biotechnology are essential parts of one framework, the person. Our justification for this assertion is directly derived from the Relational*Act*, the "acting" in life: Acting is always in one framework — it is always a *person* doing heart transplantation surgery and a *person* receiving a heart transplantation.

CHAPTER 5
*PERSON*ALIZING BIOMEDICAL RESEARCH

<table>
<tr>
<td>Ma poi ch'i' fui al piè d'un colle giunto,</td>
<td>But once I had drawn near</td>
</tr>
<tr>
<td>là dove terminava quella valle</td>
<td>the bottom of a hill at the far remove,</td>
</tr>
<tr>
<td>che m'avea di paura il cor compunto,</td>
<td>15 of the valley that had pierced my heart in fear,</td>
</tr>
<tr>
<td>guardai in alto e vidi le sue spalle</td>
<td>I saw its shoulders mantled from above,</td>
</tr>
<tr>
<td>vestite già de' raggi del pianeta</td>
<td>by the warm rays of the planet that gives light</td>
</tr>
<tr>
<td>che mena dritto altrui per ogne calle.</td>
<td>18 to guide our steps, wherever we may rove.</td>
</tr>
<tr>
<td>Allor fu la paura un poco queta,</td>
<td>At last I felt some calming of the fright</td>
</tr>
<tr>
<td>che nel lago del cor m'era durata</td>
<td>that had allowed the lake of my heart no rest</td>
</tr>
<tr>
<td>la notte ch'i' passai con tanta pieta.</td>
<td>21 while I endured the long and piteous night.</td>
</tr>
<tr>
<td>E come quei che con lena affannata,</td>
<td>And as a drowning man with heaving chest</td>
</tr>
<tr>
<td>uscito fuor del pelago a la riva,</td>
<td>escapes the current and, once safe on shore,</td>
</tr>
<tr>
<td>si volge a l'acqua perigliosa e guata,</td>
<td>24 to see the dangers he has passed,</td>
</tr>
<tr>
<td>così l'animo mio, ch'ancor fuggiva,</td>
<td>so did my mind, still lost in flight, once more</td>
</tr>
<tr>
<td>si volse a retro a rimirar lo passo</td>
<td>turn back to see the passage that had never</td>
</tr>
<tr>
<td>che non lasciò già mai persona viva.</td>
<td>27 let anyone escape alive before.</td>
</tr>
</table>

In reading these verses in Chapter 1, we wrote: "... *Imagine Dante guided by such wisdom turning toward the flickering light and discovering that its source is a laboratory light: 'Uhmm, they are testing my blood. They will know all about me, right down to my genes! I wait here. I wait for them to tell me who I am!' No need to write another canto of the Divine Comedy. There is no messy path of becoming, deference to knowledge is required.*"

We ironized a mechanistic concept of medicine that is based on the idea of establishing a linear causal relationship between genes (or proteins, cells, organs) and personhood, as an illusion creating false hope. What then is a meaningful way of addressing the relationship between the person level and the different body levels — organs, tissues, proteins and genes? The relevance of this question is as important in the medical encounters between people with different knowledge (e.g., doctor and patient) as it is in clinical and translational biomedical research. For example, what relations do exist, between the heart transplantation rejection process and the heart transplant patient experience?

Let us follow the conversation between Dr. D and Ms. Kizer in the *out*patient heart transplantation clinic examination room. Ms. Kizer underwent heart transplantation two months ago.

Ms. Kizer is a 55 year-old woman with a genetic mutation that led to production of a protein called amyloid, deposited in all body organs. After she was diagnosed, she had to undergo liver transplantation while her heart condition was still considered too stable for heart transplantation. She continued taking care of her family and working in a high stress job as a lawyer for years. Five years later, her heart condition deteriorated, requiring listing for heart transplantation. Ms. Kizer underwent heart transplantation two months prior to this encounter after having spent three months in the hospital waiting for a transplant in the high urgency category UNOS 1B.

Ms. Kizer and Dr. D are discussing the possible complication from heart transplantation rejection monitoring (biopsy, lines 24–44) and the effect of immunosuppressant medications for preventing and treating rejection (line 46).

19	Dr. D:	So, the echocardiogram,
20		you haven't had it yet?
21	Ms. Kizer:	No, haven't had yet.
22		Do I have to have one today?
23	Dr. D:	Yes, for different reasons.
24		One, after every biopsy we do an echocardiogram
25		because for every biopsy
26		there's like a 1% chance (1.9 s)
27		if you haven't had a pericardial effusion
28		that you now have one just because
29	Ms. Kizer:	Hm hm.
30	Dr. D:	this bioptome (1 s)
31		you saw this thing right?
32	Ms. Kizer:	Hm hm, yes.
33	Dr. D:	It's flexible but it's not like
34		it's not like a you know a piece of clothes.
35		It has some resistance. (1 s)
36		And the right ventricle is always
37		it's a small wall (2 s)
38		and theoretically that's why perforation
39		from a biopsy
40	Ms. Kizer:	Uhm uhm.

41	Dr. D:	is a 0.5% to
42		1.5 % chance.
43		And that's why we do echocardiogram just routinely afterwards
44		and in addition everyone is curious you know how their trends are.
45	Ms. Kizer:	That's good.
46		I have to see what my, you know,
47		for a while there, my hand was shaking wildly.
48	Dr. D:	Uhm uhm.
49	Ms. Kizer:	And I remembered it's the prograf thing.
50	Dr. D:	Uhm uhm.
51	Ms. Kizer:	I called up and it was 17 and went down to 11.
52		You I think cut back the prograf thing.
53		I just wanted to make sure it's still in a therapeutic range.
54	Dr. D:	Sure, sure.
55	Ms. Kizer:	But I need to tell you when it was working.
56		I couldn't have written a note.
57		I was trying to write thank you notes and
58		I had cross-I's and wobbly and they looked terrible!
59	Dr. D:	Yes
60	Ms. Kizer:	Terrible!
61	Dr. D:	Yea that'll be the expectations that let's say
62		the first 6 months kind of is going down.

In the dialogue above, both patient and doctor refer to procedures and use terms that we did not discuss yet in detail in this book but summarized in a brief description in Chapter 1 (Option 3). These medical procedures and treatments are now shared knowledge between Dr. D and Ms. Kizer. To understand their dialogue, we need to develop a similar framework in which these words (rejection, biopsy, echocardiogram, immunosuppressants, bioptome, perforation, crossed i's and wobbly) can develop a meaning in the context of the medical encounter of advanced heart failure and in which they are being defined as relevant.

Definitions of Heart Transplantation Rejection

Cardiac allograft rejection is the rejection of the transplanted donor heart by the heart transplant recipient, the patient. It is accepted as a process whereby the transplant recipient's immune system recognizes the cardiac allograft (transplanted heart) as a foreign body, as potentially dangerous, and tries to destroy it. In using again the mythological figure of *Janus bifrons* as discussed by Bruno Latour (1987), a procedure that has become a standard of care as heart transplantation surgery has, an understanding of a process such as rejection described above can be thought of as being looked at by one *Janus' face* gazing into what is known, what has become common practice, a black box: there is no controversy on the general understanding of the evolutionary process of allograft rejection. Yet, as Latour describes, the *Janus's* face gazing into the unknown considers that "enough is never enough" (Latour, 1987, p. 13). In advanced heart failure biomedical research, this *Janus'* face gazes into the relevant definitions of rejection for developing diagnostic and therapeutic interventions.

Cardiac allograft rejection can be defined in the conceptual frameworks of different biomedical fields and methods of investigation.

In molecular immunology, it is understood as a molecular–immunological process. The immune cells of the recipient (transplanted patient) recognize the donor heart as foreign and therefore dangerous for the body. The molecules on the donor heart cell surface (allo-antigens) trigger the heart transplant patient's white blood cells' immune response (T-cell-mediated) to destroy all the cells of the allograft (donor heart).

At a tissue-level (histology), the process of allograft rejection is understood as the presence of immune cells such as T-cells in the allograft tissue. Their presence is interpreted as having the function (pathological process) of destroying the allograft (transplanted donor heart). The histological process of rejection — diagnosed by endomyocardial biopsy — is studied by taking three to six one-millimeter-size pieces from the allograft, the transplanted heart of the transplanted patient.

At the organ level, rejection is understood as an impairment of the organ's function of pumping blood to the body (pathophysiological process of allograft dysfunction). Heart ultrasound, electrocardiogram and right heart catheter are used together to detect organ dysfunction related to rejection.

At the person level (clinical), rejection is understood as process of symptomatic heart failure and death.

Each of these definitions emphasizes a different discipline's viewpoint on the heart transplantation rejection process: molecular immunology, pathology, pathophysiology, and clinical medicine.

Do any of these rejection concepts deserve primacy over the other ones in clinical and translational research and patient care? The answer depends on the perspective and background that a clinician or researcher is taking. Each of these definitions, by emphasizing a different conceptual aspect of the rejection process, is at the same time abstracting from the other aspects of the rejection process. In the journal *Current Opinion in Organ Transplantation*, Deng, Cadeiras and Reed (2013) capture what they call *the multidimensional perspective of cardiac allograft rejection* by recollecting the metaphor of the four blind men who attempt to define the 'Gestalt' of an elephant, each of the four blind men claiming 'to know how the elephant looks', each of them capturing a different, yet important aspect of the elephant — the trunk, the ears, the belly, and the legs. As they write in their editorial: "Any solution to the question, whether one concept deserves primacy over the other concept, needs to start with a reflection on the representatives of the four concepts — let us call them the molecular immunologist, the pathologist, the pathophysiologist, and the clinician — about their individual processes of respective abstraction decisions that each of them have made in their concept development process" (p. 569) (See also Figure 5.1).

Endomyocardial biopsy defined rejection

With its development in 1973, endomyocardial biopsy, producing results on the tissue level perceived as more accurate than the electrocardiogram,

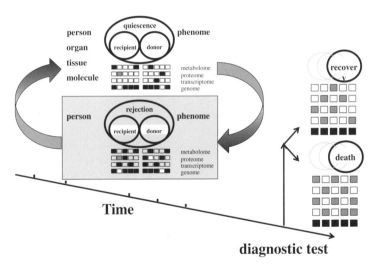

Figure 5.1: Tests for diagnosing and predicting heart transplantation rejection and absence of rejection (quiescence) and their consequences (recovery or death) can be defined on different biomedical levels including (1) *person* level or clinical (phenome), (2) organ function level (pathophysiology), (3) tissue level, for example as assessed by biopsy (pathology), or (4) molecular level (including genome, transcriptome, proteome, metabolome) (modified after Deng, Cadeiras and Reed, 2013, details see text).

echocardiogram and clinical assessment, has become the standard diagnostic test worldwide to detect heart transplantation rejection. With this new tool for diagnosis, histology has become the gold standard to define heart transplantation rejection (Deng, 2010).

The endomyocardial biopsy method, also referred to as heart muscle biopsy or among advanced heart failure healthcare professionals, patients and their families simply as 'biopsy', as in Dr. D's and Ms. Kizer's encounter, requires the patient to have a procedure in the catheter lab, while lying flat on the catheter table under a sterile cloth (Figure 5.2). The patient is often covered completely, that is, most often the face is also hidden by a sterile cloth. The biopsy is performed by the advanced heart failure cardiologist.

The procedure can take from 15 to 60 minutes depending on the difficulty and complexity of each single case. It comprises the following steps, each with its difficulties and potential for complications.

(1) Locating the neck vein: Classically, the technique to locate the neck vein consists of identifying an anatomical landmark such as the lateral

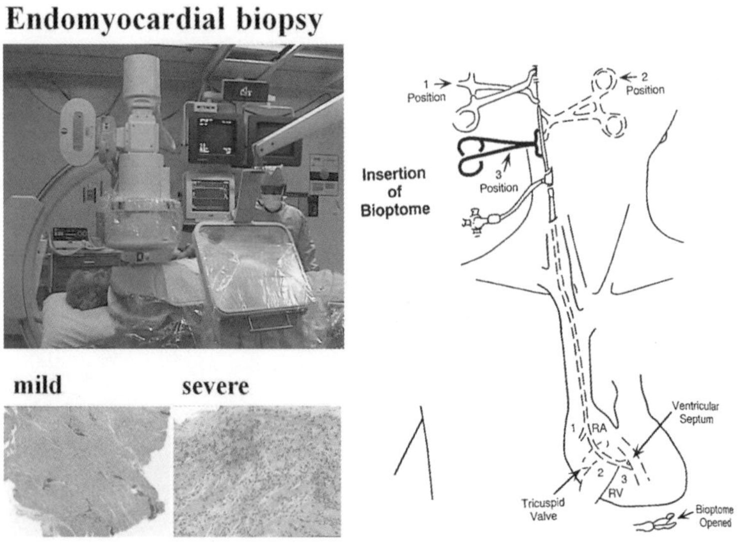

Endomyocardial biopsy

Figure 5.2: Endomyocardial biopsy: Patient lying on catheter lab table (upper left), bioptome inserted into right internal jugular vein to remove heart muscle specimens from right ventricular heart muscle (right), histological diagnosis of heart transplant rejection (lower left)(details see text).

sternocleidomastoideus muscle belly boundary by asking the patient, who is lying on the catheter table and under the cloth, to turn her/his head to the left side and then raise the head. By doing so, the patient's neck muscle contracts and demarcates the lateral boundary of the muscle. This boundary area forms the entry site for the local anesthesia needle and the subsequent finder needle to place the guide-wire in the vein. In using the anatomical landmark method, difficulties can arise in locating the vein precisely. A difficulty can arise for example from the presence of scar tissue in the skin or in the vein wall of the patient after repeated biopsies. Other difficulties of locating the vein can arise from the higher doses of diuretics that patients often need to take, causing low blood volume status in the patient's body and a small diameter of the collapsed vein. These difficulties may lead to prolonged times in the procedure of placing the guide-wire and is associated with varying degrees of discomfort and/or pain for the patient. Under such circumstances, there is an increased risk for one of the complications of endomyocardial biopsy — the accidental puncture of the carotid artery. This artery that runs directly adjacent to the neck vein carries blood with high pressure, so, if punctured, a fast flow of blood can rush into the surrounding tissue with subsequent large hematoma formation. An improved method in identifying a patient's vein is using ultrasound guidance prior to or while placing the local anesthesia.

Dr. D in CoGen reflects: "For some physicians, being able to find the vein without the aid of ultrasound has unfortunately been a source of pride. Resorting to ultrasound only after having been poking the patient's neck for several minutes, has a higher chance to produce complications and more pain for the patient, augmenting a sense of being an object under the cloth and sense of uncertainty about the process."

Mr. Stafford is a 56 year-old man with non-ischemic cardiomyopathy of sudden onset, likely from a viral myocarditis-induced inflammatory heart muscle disease, for which he underwent successful heart transplantation. Two months later, after a painful endomyocardial biopsy, he recounts:

> It is not easy to be there. You feel like an object. They are operating on you and you don't see anything, but you think, well it has to be done. You lie

there and it is not easy to say hey wait! Something is wrong! I am in pain and it feels a different pain, something is wrong. You lie there, you just do not think to say anything.

(2) The placement of the guide wire: After having introduced the finder needle — the needle to find the vein — into the vein, a wire of a diameter that is a fraction of a millimeter known as the guide wire is advanced through the finder needle into the vein. If the vein is partially occluded from previous intravascular clot formation, the advancement of the wire may be difficult and require fluoroscopic (X-ray) guidance. If the advancement of the wire is difficult, the patient feels the thrusting of the guide wire and the resistance to it. This maneuvering is often accompanied by conversations between the healthcare professionals about the procedure. From being an object under the cloth, new anxieties about the uncertainty of the process and the outcome of the biopsy beset the patient: What if they cannot get a piece of the heart to see if I have rejection?

(3) Sheath placement: When the guide wire is successfully placed in the vein, the finder needle is removed and a dilator, introduced over the guide wire, is used to dilate the vein to create a conduit to place a 2–3 millimeter diameter and 15 centimeter long sheath in the vein. The sheath serves as the conduit for the subsequent placement of the bioptome (as shown in Figure 5.2), introduced over the guide wire into the vein. The time required for this part of the endomyocardial biopsy procedure may vary because the continuous scarring of the skin and vein wall from repeated biopsy trauma may lead to obstruction for the sheath placement. At times, the physician doing the biopsy needs to apply various degrees of force to overcome the obstruction and penetrate the vein. This is a very delicate situation because being told to "bear down" (see transcript of patient Ms. Kizer below) or be patient in a situation where one is lying down on the catheter table covered by a cloth to keep the wound sterile, with needles, tubes, bioptome in the body and being worked on by others makes a person feel even more powerless than he/she already does: "you lie there, you just do not think to say anyting". The patient in that moment is the patient's body, an object and not in full possession of her/his *person*hood.

Ms. Kizer recounts with Dr. D the right heart catheterization procedure that was performed before her placement on the UNOS 1B waiting list, 93 days prior to transplantation:

Ms. Kizer: But but but ... In order to take the heart tissue samples you've gotta come in here right?
It's only ...
It sounds so stupid ...
Just find someone who is really good at it ...
Who has done it a lot of times ...
I came out with a little bruise and it hurt ...
I am happy if you wanna put me to sleep ...
Give me something ... but
I lie down ...
My head is down ...
For one I don't have very much blood ...
You know I think the only thing he said to me [was] "bear down" ...
Right now ... god knows what he was doing ...
Okay I don't bear down unless I get a baby to take home ...
Explain to me why it is ... you know what I mean ...
I didn't understand what the problem was ... well
I sort of understand it I did not have enough blood ...
anything like that ...
You know and ...
of course it took him a number of times to
You know ...
I don't have much of ...
I know this is a teaching hospital ...

(4) Bioptome introduction: Once the sheath is in place, the bioptome, a flexible catheter with scissors at the tip (Figure 5.2), is advanced through it into the vein, then advanced under fluoroscopic (X-ray) guidance into the right side of the heart. To enter into the right ventricle, the bioptome passes through the right atrium of the heart and the tricuspid valve that separates the right atrium and right ventricle. This is a delicate passage because of the anatomy of the tricuspid valve, which can be damaged. This complication produces tricuspid regurgitation, which can lead to right heart failure of the transplant heart.

(5) Biopsy specimen sampling: The bioptome is then advanced towards the interventricular septum, the heart muscle wall that separates the right and the left ventricle of the heart, and three to six pieces of heart muscle, each 1–2 cubic millimeter in size, are removed. The insertion of

the bioptome into the heart can produce potentially dangerous irregular fast heartbeats (arrhythmias).

This biopsy procedure, if the right jugular vein is not feasible for access, can alternatively be carried out through the left jugular vein or either of the femoral (groin) veins, in which case the procedure may take longer.

91	Dr. D:	I have been doing biopsy for 25 years now
92		and it is something that every time
93		the situation takes place, I in a way feel like
94		if I were lying on a table
95		I would not like it.
96		I would try to do my best but
97		I would not look forward to it.
98	Ms. Kizer:	To me the nurse
99		just to start,
100		takes my hands.
101		Her hands are so warm and
102		I've said it before but
103		it's like good medicine you know (1.2 s)
104		to feel another human being, someone supporting you
105		someone with you.
106		Just, it's . . . It's so powerful.
107	Dr. D:	Uhm uhm.
108	Ms. Kizer:	and I know that she is already in there
109		so you know it doesn't take any extra time,
110	Dr. D:	Uhm uhm.
111	Ms. Kizer:	but you feel less like an object or a patient
112		and much more like
113		you're with people who are going to take care of you.
114	Dr. D:	Uhm uhm.
115	Ms. Kizer:	So I have to say she is just,
116		she is the only person I've seen done this.
117		Really.
118	Dr. D:	Interesting.
119		Yes.
120		It's so important.
121	Ms. Kizer:	It really is.
122		You can't see anybody (1 s).
123	Dr. D:	Yes it's so important.
124	Ms. Kizer:	Yes!
125	Dr. D:	It's at the core
126		I think it's really important at [hospital name]
127		a biopsy suite nurse
128		is like the soul you know.

129		Every good program has someone like a soul you know.
130		There is a person or persons who are
131		beyond kind of the average working day
132		and, you know the typical thing, good
133		and are personally available as persons and
134		if you ask anyone who has been at [hospital name]
135		you know having had biopsies there she is there.
136		You can't even explain that to someone who doesn't get it
137		why it's a good idea if
138		if I'm lying there as a patient to just hold my hand.
139		It's rational . . .
140		If you do it rational but you don't feel it,
141		it doesn't really help actually.
142	Ms. Kizer:	Yea I can feel her like
143		when I'm squeezing she is squeezing back.
144		In the other lab the nurse just holding my hands . . .
145	Dr. D:	I think it's beautiful.
146	Ms. Kizer:	When it hurts
147		I go like this
148		she just you know and she doesn't say a word but
149		It's so like a really good pain reliever sedative.

As we describe below, the biopsy protocol is carried out with varied frequency after heart transplantation. After having had several biopsies, a patient's allograft heart may have scars formed in the small area on the right side of the interventricular septum to which the bioptome has access. The repeated search for the sampling sites in the heart increases the chance of one of the most feared complications: the perforation of the right ventricular wall with pericardial tamponade (pericardial effusion) with an overall incidence of 0.5–1.5%.

When the perforation is caused by the bioptome, the blood leaves the inside of the heart and flows into the space between the heart and the surrounding pericardial sac. This may impede the filling of the heart with blood and may require an urgent rescue therapy by either catheter insertion into the pericardial sac to remove the blood or emergency surgery with reopening of the chest to remove the pericardial blood. Note that pericardial tamponade may be caused not only by a biopsy complication but also by other conditions. For example, it can result as a complication after any open heart surgery, as was suspected for Ms. Loy (Chapter 4) following heart transplantation.

The pieces collected by the bioptome are further processed, cut into thin sections, stained, viewed under the microscope with the goal of identifying areas of heart muscle with white blood cell infiltration and heart muscle damage, as shown on the lower left side of Figure 5.2.

The biopsy protocol is being used by all 300 heart transplantation centers in the world and varies slightly in frequency.

In the university hospital center where Dr. D works, the biopsy protocol has a specific schedule based on clinical research data of expected likelihood of rejection after heart transplantation. As Dr. D presented in both the Patient Education Seminar at the hospital where he works and at various Advanced Heart Failure symposia (Figure 5.3), a biopsy is performed every week for the first four weeks after transplantation surgery. Starting on week six, it is performed every two weeks until the end of the second month post-transplantation (indicated with a dark grey area in Figure 5.3). From month three post-transplantation, the biopsy is performed each month until the end of month six post-transplantation. In the second half year post-transplantation, between months seven and twelve, the biopsy is performed

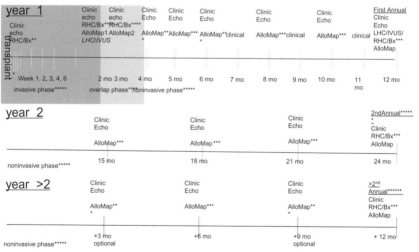

Figure 5.3: UCLA heart transplantation rejection monitoring protocol.

every two months. From year two post-transplantation, the default protocol provides that the biopsy is performed every three (to six) months.

In addition to the biopsy protocol utilized in a hospital, a biopsy is performed whenever heart transplant rejection is suspected.

The biopsy results are reported as graded by the consensus classification of the International Society for Heart and Lung Transplantation as grade 0 (no rejection = quiescence), 1R = mild rejection, 2R = moderate rejection, and 3R = severe rejection. If rejection of grades 2R or 3R are indicated, immunosuppression is increased for several days, followed by another biopsy.

Because the endomyocardial biopsy captures only a late stage aspect of rejection that may not easily be reversible, the increase in immunosuppression dose usually includes, as part of a three drug immunosuppression protocol, the increase of the steroid hormone prednisone by a factor of 100 to a dose of 500–1000 mg/day over three days. This dose is 50–100 times higher than the usual amount produced and required by the body, and has many side effects, including increased susceptibility to (1) infection, (2) diabetes, (3) osteoporosis, (4) psychiatric symptoms varying from mood swings to psychosis, (5) high blood pressure, and (6) high blood lipid levels.

Based on the risks associated with the biopsy procedure, the limits of the information rendered, its invasive nature and the painful and potentially distressing experience for the patient, over the last 25 years there have been many attempts to develop alternative methods to diagnose or rule out heart transplant rejection. While efforts toward finding alternative tests (that are less painful, cause less complications, capture earlier stages of rejection that may be more easily reversible, and are less expensive) were made, none of the non-invasive methods developed were successful until some years ago. As none of these tests met the performance characteristics to replace the endomyocardial biopsy, biopsy remained the gold standard procedure to detect rejection in all heart transplantation centers in the world.

In 2006, Dr. D, in a large collaborative research study called 'Cardiac Allograft Rejection Gene-expression Observation (CARGO) Study' (Deng *et al.*, 2006), showed that a new blood test based on the revolutionary sequencing of the Human Genome in 2001 (Venter *et al.*, 2001) and revolutionary new technology allowing for high-throughput gene-expression profiling via DNA-microarray technology, could be used to rule out heart transplantation rejection in stable heart transplantation patients without the need for routine endomyocardial biopsy. As a byproduct of this study, the CARGO investigator team showed that, by tissue (histology)-based rejection diagnosis using the endomyocardial biopsy, there are up to 50% false positive acute cardiac allograft rejection episodes diagnosed, leading to unnecessary overtreatment with high doses of steroid hormones.

Leukocyte expression profile and rejection

The CARGO study was initiated in the year 2000 as a collaboration among four large US academic heart transplant centers and was soon thereafter joined by four other major US academic heart transplant centers. The project goal was to develop a peripheral white blood cell (leukocyte) test to rule out rejection, termed the Allomap™ test (Deng *et al.*, 2006). The team hypothesized that a novel diagnostic strategy could be developed to better monitor rejection than the standard of care based on protocol endomyocardial biopsy. The research team started from the following basic idea, as Dr. D discusses with his patients, and describes in CoGen: "If I have a transplanted heart from another person, my white blood cells continuously travel with my blood stream into the transplanted heart's vessels and get into direct contact with the other person's vessel lining cells, the endothelial cells. During this continuous interaction between my white blood cells (leukocytes) and the other person's endothelial cells in the transplanted heart (allograft), a fight is taking place. If my white blood cells detect 'danger', they enter the muscle of the transplanted heart".

As we discussed above, this would be the aspect of the rejection process as the biopsy would capture; but these cells, as Dr. D continues his explanation, "produce/release protein molecules that have the goal of destroying the transplanted heart's cells. Some of my white blood cells, in their journey in the blood stream of my vessels, leave the transplanted heart and flow with the blood stream, returning into my peripheral blood vessels, for example my arm veins. Now, how about if I can just ask my leuokocytes, my white blood cells, in my peripheral blood: 'What did you guys see when you were in the transplanted heart? Was there any problem with the other person's heart cells trying to attack us?' If the leukocytes contain the information about rejection or absence of rejection in the transplanted heart, we elegantly get this information, for example by understanding varying activity patterns of gene expression of the thousands of genes that make a white blood cell 'tick', without having to take pieces out of my transplanted heart, without biopsy, non-invasively. This would allow a patient with heart transplant to have a less painful, safer, and potentially less costly test."

The question we now raise is how a research project and a test development such as Allomap can play an important role in *person*alizing modern medicine.

Here we provide a biomedical research summary of the Allomap test development to understand how, from the research perspective, the concept of personalizing medicine enters into the discussion and what role it plays in high-tech modern medicine.

The Allomap test is a test measuring the combined activity of 11 indicator genes (genes that had been identified in the process of the Allomap test development) in a subpopulation of our white blood cells circulating through the vessels of our body (as traffic police officers looking out for traffic violators, so to speak) called peripheral blood mononuclear cells (PBMC), correlated with the absence of rejection. The gene activity is translated into a sum score, arbitrarily scaled from 1–39, with 39 indicating a higher likelihood of the presence of acute cellular cardiac allograft rejection. Since the Allomap score, in comparison to the biopsy score with four categories, contains a scale of 39 categories, it can provide a finer granular reflection of the rejection process.

The Allomap test development in the original CARGO study, the CARGO I Study (Deng *et al.*, 2006), led to clinical implementation in the year 2006 (Starling *et al.*, 2006) and the clearance of this first in history molecular rejection blood test by the US Food and Drug Administration (FDA) in 2008. The European CARGO II Study confirmed the performance characteristics in the European heart transplant recipient cohort (Crespo-Leiro *et al.*, 2009). As an additional validation study, the "Invasive Monitoring Attenuation by GeneExpression" (IMAGE) Study was conducted, hypothesizing that an integrated non-invasive diagnostic strategy was not worse than (non-inferior to) endomyocardial biopsy-based monitoring in detecting clinically relevant rejection, combined with improved patient satisfaction (Pham *et al.*, 2010).

A step towards personalizing medicine

The ongoing research on the clinical application of Allomap is showing how the test, beyond concurrent episodes of rejection, also has an application in predicting future events of rejection if more than one Allomap score of a patient is analyzed over time. The lower the variability of the Allomap score over time, the lower the likelihood of developing a clinically relevant rejection event. That is, the test helped in establishing a clinical impression of absence of rejection for Mr. James, Ms. Loy, Mr. Montale, Ms. Mereau, Mr. Phillip, Mr. Alcman, Mr. Carroll, Ms. Grahn, and Ms. Kizer. Their individual biology and, therefore, their clinical stories, each with its own specific clinical individuality, were different from the stories of the other patients, the other *persons*. This further test development of longitudinal time-series leukocyte gene expression profiling after regulatory approval of the Allomap test concept introduces a completely novel criterion, i.e., long-term gene expression variability as a predictor of relevant clinical rejection events (Deng *et al.*, 2014).

Non-Invasive Rejection Monitoring in the Clinical Encounter

From the perspective of a heart transplant recipient, the question is whether the Allomap test fulfills my expectations of being the most effective, safe, and reliable method.

Here it is important to underline a fundamental transformation that has implications in the practice of high-tech modern medicine.

As described above, the development and the implementation of the Allomap test has shown that the endomyocardial biopsy diagnoses up to 50% false positive acute cardiac allograft rejection episodes and that more levels of information are required to optimally monitor stable heart transplantation recipients for rejection. This suggests that monitoring a heart transplantation patient for rejection is a complex process requiring multilevel information: It implies that the blind man knowing the molecular immunology (transcriptome = gene expression profiling) level, the molecular immunologist, should link into the definition of the two other blind men, i.e., the clinician who knows the clinical signs and symptoms of rejection and the pathophysiologist who knows the organ function signs of rejection. These levels all carry important and complementary information about the patient, and, therefore, need to be integrated at the person level during the medical encounter.

This approach requires, on the part of the patient, attentive and active monitoring for clinical signs such as palpitations and water retention, as well as the symptoms of shortness of breath and fatigue. In fact, this modern rejection monitoring approach, using the high-technology research products, requires a more active, agency-claiming patient involvement. It suggests that patient and caregiver education needs to emphasize the importance of self-monitoring for signs and symptoms, specifically since the old standard of biopsy, being unchallenged for more than thirty years, wrongfully suggested that physician and patient should rely almost exclusively on the presence or absence of sign of rejection as defined by histology. Wrongfully, because even in the biopsy era, if you did a protocol biopsy, from year 1 on, every 3 months, and even if you assume that the biopsy gives information for the following 7 days, you would be without histology information for a period of 90 days − 7days = 83 days, or 90% of the time. During this 90% of the time, the decision-making would follow clinical (and not histology) criteria, i.e., signs and symptoms (person-level) as well as new onset graft dysfunction (organ function level) in the absence of a third validated level of information that now is provided by the Allomap testing concept.

As Dr. D explains to his patients: "If you feel well and you can do anything you want to do in daily life and your transplant heart is pumping well on heart ultrasound then all that is happening at the level of histology/pathology cannot be that bad."

In stable heart transplantation patients, serial non-invasive monitoring with Allomap can safely achieve down-dosing of immunosuppressive medication, for example by monthly monitoring of both Allomap and heart function during the clinical encounter. This requires active participation of patient and family caregiver as discussants in the regulation of immunosuppressants.

The explicit relationship between three system levels is new: gene, organ and *person* level. All are taken into consideration at the same time.

The less invasive and less painful procedure, as the blood draw for advanced heart failure patients represents, also alleviates the anxiety of heart transplant patients over the upcoming painful biopsy procedure.

A more satisfying rejection monitoring concept also has implications for supporting younger, for example adolescent, patients in maintaining rejection monitoring follow-up appointments instead of, at times, missing appointments for fear of undergoing a biopsy procedure.

All these advantages of the Allomap-based monitoring concept prepare the ground to individualize/personalize the heart transplantation follow-up in the iterative encounter sequence between healthcare professional and patient. In this sense, this research-based clinical innovation is groundbreaking as it has the power to transform the medical encounter. Physicians and patients no longer rely almost exclusively on the presence or absence of signs of rejection as defined by histology. In contrast, the questions that Dr. D asks himself during the encounter *preparation phase* are: Is my patient clinically stable. i.e., has no signs and symptoms of rejection? Does my patient have normal heart transplantation graft function? These questions lead to an attunement of both, patient and physician, to the patient's perception of body signs and symptoms. This *person*-level information shared during the encounter is integrated with the molecular immunological level information to provide a complementary set of information about the likelihood of presence/absence of clinically relevant rejection.

The Relational*Act* encounter between a heart transplant cardiologist and a heart transplant patient who is eligible for Allomap monitoring could thus proceed as follows:

Today Dr. D is meeting with his patient, Ms. Kizer, who underwent heart transplantation more than two months ago, feels well and has normal heart transplantation function, to discuss the option of offering her the non-invasive, Allomap-based, heart transplantation rejection monitoring concept.

Dr. D is aware that Ms. Kizer is medically eligible since (1) the patient is more than 56 days post-transplantation (the United States Food and Drug Administration (US-FDA) allows the use of the test from Day 56 after heart transplantation); (2) the patient feels well; (3) the patient has normal heart transplantation function; and (4) the patient has had no major rejection periods on the biopsies at week 1, 2, 3, 4, and 6. In the encounter, Dr. D first reviews her eligibility, i.e., whether the patient is fulfilling the clinical criteria of stability, normal graft function and absence of recurrent dangerous rejection episodes. Next, Dr. D offers this option to his patient as we showed above. For Ms. Kizer, the non-invasive monitoring translates to the (1) safest possible evidence-based monitoring with respect to survival and transplant heart function, and (2) best possible quality of life enhancement. For Dr. D as the healthcare professional, the non-invasive monitoring provides a feeling of satisfaction that he is offering the best evidence-based clinical practices to his patient that is at the same time pain free and safe.

Thus, Dr. D, in his recursive encounters with Ms. Kizer, uses information originating from history-taking, physical examination, organ function and white blood cell biology to explore Ms. Kizer's health situation and to guide his recommendations for her. In analogy to our understanding of the encounter between healthcare professional and patient as a recursive two-person process that we have termed, the Relational*Act* the physician-philosopher Viktor von Weizsaecker, influential co-founder of the field of psychosomatic medicine posited in 1950, in his Gestaltkreis concept (*integrative process of the subject-environment relationship in the Biological Act*) that: 'To explore life, you have to participate in life. Although one can make the attempt to derive Living from Non-Living, this endeavor so far has failed. One can also try to be in denial of one's own life in the sciences, but this is doomed to be a self-deception. At the beginning of all life sciences is not the beginning of life itself, but the science has begun with the awakening of the questions in the middle of living' (1950, p. 3). Dr. D: "Only if I make sense of myself as a person, then I can participate in understanding Ms. Kizer as my patient in her person-body situation".

CHAPTER 6
CONCLUSION

We started this book by encountering Mrs. More and meeting Mr. Montale, Ms. Mereau, Ms. Grahn, Mr. Phillip, Mr. Carroll, Mr. Rice, Mr. James, Mr. Alcman, Ms. Loy, Mr. Stafford, Ms. Kizer and Dante at the onset of a journey *in medias res*, at a point, in each of their lives, from where it is impossible to continue on the same path, as all meaning of each of their worlds has collapsed: the land of dissimilitude. To start making sense of these persons' experiences in the high-tech *modern medicine* practice of advanced heart failure, we built on Dante's poetry and Heidegger's philosophical work.

Dante's poetry guided us in disclosing a sense of being lost in the land of dissimilitude at a point from where it is impossible to continue on the same path we were on. It helped us not by developing a rational understanding of it, but by *having a sense of* ourselves as human beings, dwelling in a world where death is part of life, that is, being *in medias res* at a turning point. It is a turning point not only because all that had meaning has collapsed, but because, as Dante anticipates in the first ten verses of his long journey through *Inferno*, *Purgatorio* and *Paradiso* (v. 8–9 *ma per trattar del ben ch'i' vi trovai,/dirò de l'altre cose ch'i' v'ho scorte*), it is a journey to transform a raw terrifying harsh forest (*oscura selvaggia e aspra*) into an ancient forest (*selva antica*) of lush and luxuriant foliage (*spessa e viva*). In the land of dissimilitude, all that had *significance*, has been lost. We cannot follow some formula on how to find the straight path to get out of the *selva oscura*. As our understanding of who we are is grounded in the specificity of the activities we engage in, the specificity of experiences we have in interaction with things and with others, in the specificity of the context, situation, world in which we dwell, we cannot get out of the *selva oscura*. However, we can transform it. We must transform it to recognize this life as ours. We turn to Heidegger's philosophy in *Being and Time*, as it is centered on deepening our understanding of what it means for something and somebody to be in relation to others and to things in the world. Based on his work, we understand that the two complementary experiences, *how* a person copes with equipment and other people in her/his world, and *how* this person makes sense of his/her own identity, are deeply intertwined. It is on this account that we made visible the irreducible experiences of illness and disease, as a person's world collapses in high-tech modern medicine.

A person with advanced heart failure does not see her/himself as a whole person but as one with a body which has become an instrument that has failed to do its job, with replaceable broken-down part(s), 'unready-to-hand'. These are inseparable experiences of one's own body as a broken tool and of threat to one's existence: Who I am is "a scary character in the movies, half man, half machine", "a science experiment". This is the land of dissimilitude.

There, Heidegger says, we are alone. Yes, we are, as nobody can make sense of what it means to be living with a BiVAD through the experience of another person living with it. And, most importantly, these experiences are *this* person's experiences, and it is *this* person, Mr. James for instance, who needs to integrate a BiVAD into *his* life. These experiences of interaction with high-tech modern medicine are novel to patients and their family caregivers and unknown to physicians.

The technological advancements in the experiences of Mr. James, Mr. Rice, Mr. Montale, Mr. Phillip, Mr. Alcman, Ms. Mereau, Ms. Grahn, Mr. Carroll, Ms. Loy, Mr. Stafford and Ms. Kizer and their family caregivers, hoping for life in the face of death, are experiences of high-tech modern medicine. High-tech modern medicine is forcing new territories for humans to dwell. Here, dealing with and becoming familiar with a Total Artificial Heart, with an LVAD, with a BiVAD, with the heart from somebody else, is not possible for one person alone. It requires that the one who is lost in the land of dissimilitude recognizes the Other and is recognized by the Other to transform a *selva oscura* into her/his *selva antica*. The human experience in advanced heart failure is an experience *shared with others*.

How to help a person with advanced heart failure, lost in the land of dissimilitude, and to make her/his world familiar is the concern of a healthcare professional in high-tech modern medicine.

In this book, we made visible through the study of Dr. D's practice, how a healthcare professional recognizes and helps a person with advanced heart failure operate this transformation. We grounded this *transformation* in the

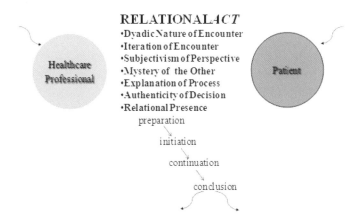

Figure 6.1: Relational*Act* (RA) encounter between healthcare professional and patient: recurring encounter aspects and encounter phases (details see text).

irreducible historicity of this person and saw the encounter process unfold as a relational process.

We made visible Dr. D's practice, as it unfolds in each encounter, as a sequence of *preparation, initiation, continuation,* and *conclusion phases.* Each medical encounter as well as each phase of the encounter builds on recurrent relational aspects, "between myself and the Other," as Dr. D puts it in Figure 6.1.

Dr. D continuously experiences each of these recurring relational aspects during every encounter in an integrated way, with varying emphasis on each of them as felt important to make sense of the encounter in a given moment. We have seen, for example, his own *relational presence* in being silent for 20 seconds with Mrs. More as she is developing an understanding that her husband is dying. We have seen, for example, how important it is for Dr. D to learn about his patient's experience and attune to where the patient is in his/her journey of transformation (*iteration of the encounter*) as he does, for example, with Ms. Loy and Mr. James. We also have seen how in helping a patient, Mr. James, in following his regimen to recovery, Dr. D takes Mr. James' complaint about pain as the irreducible starting point (*mystery of the Other*). In Dr. D's framework, Mr. James' pain represents a two-fold challenge, a physical impediment that needs to be addressed *and* as a signal that perhaps Mr. James is lost in the land of dissimilitude. In advanced heart failure if Mr. James concentrates exclusively on a part of his body in pain (unready-to-hand), this body part becomes *obtrusive* in his experience of living with the (*obstinate*) machine. This would preclude possibilities for Mr. James' to operate a transformation that is needed for his survival. Dr. D needs to create a meaningful path together with Mr. James to start making this transformation. This is possible as Mr. James and Dr. D create a safe space in which temporality of Mr. James' experience is integrated as his relational past and his future possibilities are constitutive parts of Mr. James' present transformation. During the encounter, this manifests in the synchronization of perspectives: two persons acting within the same framework, reciprocally relating to one another (*dyadism*).

This space for a patient's life's transformations toward *agency*, towards owning one's life's decisions, is possible (*authenticity of decision*), it is one where walking, sitting, eating, talking, working, being a father, a nurse, a teacher etc., can become integrated into the new *way of being familiar* with an LVAD, with a BiVAD, with a Total Artificial Heart or with a transplant heart. We have seen how this has to be subtle. For example, the translation of Mr. James' words (of being with a BiVAD) 'weird', into a 'big thing' is subtle. A 'big thing', since the BiVAD implantation transforms Mr. James' own *obtrusive* body into a victorious body in his fight against death; a transformation from the body as malfunctioning equipment with broken parts, *Unzuhandenheit/unready-to-hand*, (Heidegger, 1927/1962) into a person-level achievement. A subtle translation that can be used by the patient to start the transformation: 'Yes it's a big thing!' Mr. James says. Doctor and patient accomplish this together. A transformation is also necessary for the physician as we see in the encounter with Ms. Loy. Dr. D operates a transformation for himself in order to make sense of Ms. Loy's difficulties in dealing with a heart transplantation process with two preceding dry runs, in order to continue to properly care for her.

The transformations in high-tech modern medicine require translations of questions from the world of science and scientific-technological interventions, dealing with natural functions, termed by Heidegger *Zuhandenheit/present-at hand* (1927/1962), into questions of what these mean on *this person's* level. In the encounter we see the *explanation of the process* always given in the context where it is part of the patient's and his/her family's experience. In any given specific moment and in *this* patient's and family's experience, the function of this explanation is always to support the transformation of *selva oscura* into *selva antica*.

It is in the practice of high-tech modern medicine as we see it enacted in advanced heart failure, that it is possible for a doctor to recognize a patient in the *selva oscura*. In the obtrusiveness of all that has broken down in this patient's life, the healthcare professional can help this person start making sense in his/her life, start coping with things in the world in his/her own way as the world starts becoming familiar again to the patient. In this process, her/his transforming identity becomes recognizable to her/himself.

In this act, what the Relational Medicine practice of high-tech modern medicine means is experienced not only by the patient but also by Dr. D. What it means for him to be a doctor, to *do* medicine, is now grounded in making possible the necessary transformation which his patients need to *do* in the land of dissimilitude, from *selva oscura* to *selva antica*.

It is this act in high-tech modern medicine that is a Relational*Act*.

O luce etterna che sola in te sidi,	O Light Eternal that alone abitest thyself, alone
sola t'intendi, e da te intelletta	knowest thyself, and, known to thyself.
e intendente te ami e arridi!	126 And knowing, lovest and smilest on thyself!
Quella circulazion che sì concetta	That circling which, thus begotten,
pareva in te come lume reflesso,	appeared in thee as reflected light.
da li occhi miei alquanto circunspetta,	When mine eyes dwelt on it for a time,
dentro da sé, del suo colore stesso,	seem to me within it and its own itself color,
mi parve pinta de la nostra effige:	painted with our likeness, for which
per che 'l mio viso in lei tutto era messo.	my sight was wholly given to it.

And Dante, in his journey from the land of dissimilitude to the last canto of Paradise, awed by the vision of the eternal light, in it recognizes *himself.*

AFTERWORD

As healthcare in the United States continues to undergo profound change, many academic health centers, like the UCLA Health System, have embarked on a course of innovation and revitalization. Our leadership, faculty, and staff all understand that in order to flourish in this new landscape, we must make fundamental changes in the way we provide care.

Focusing on patients is paramount among these shifts. In the past, academic health centers were often built and operated to meet the needs of clinical research and training. However, in this new world of value, systems must focus more on patients – their needs, their values, and their preferences. When patients are at the core, driving clinical decisions, they are the ones who define the importance and quality of their healthcare experience.

In tackling this crucial task of developing more patient-focused models of care (integrated approaches that follow the patient in the environment of a high-tech, tertiary and quaternary academic health center), the patient's perspective needs to be better understood. To accomplish this task we need to develop research methods that allow us to follow the patient, capturing the encounter between patient, caregiver and healthcare professional when and where it is happening.

The Relational*Act* Model research method and the Relational*Act* clinical care concept that was developed by UCLA Professors Federica Raia and Mario Deng is a fine example of such an innovative, patient-focused approach. The goal of their work closely parallels that of the Patient Centered Outcomes Research Institute (PCORI) that was created by the Affordable Care Act. I know PCORI well, having served as the founding chair of its Board of Governors. PCORI's mission is to fund and promote evidence-based research that ultimately will help patients make informed healthcare decisions and thus improve healthcare delivery and outcomes. This imperative is based on the vision that patients and the public need to have the full breadth of information that research can provide in order to make decisions that reflect their desired health outcomes.

A second key element critical to re-inventing academic medicine is the need to reorganize our health centers so that we deliver care in a value-conscious mode. How can we assess the value associated with different therapeutic options in a specific situation for a specific patient? We must go beyond the immediate patient encounter to capture outcomes in quality of life and resumption of everyday activities.

Professors Raia and Deng's new work, which explores "the practice of high-tech medicine as a Relational*Act*," lays out an excellent roadmap for change, an approach to implementing these essential innovations in healthcare. None of us in academic medicine can afford to sit on the sidelines as our world changes. This book is a significant contribution in offering solutions to meet the nation's enormous and evolving healthcare needs.

A. Eugene Washington, MD, MSc
Vice Chancellor of UCLA Health Sciences
Dean of the David Geffen School of Medicine at UCLA

I cried while reading the first paragraphs of the Introduction to this book. I was there with you, Dr. Raia, as you so artfully and accurately captured the power of the situation, observing Dr. Deng leading the team, caring for the very sick patient and the family that loved him. I was there in the moment with you and in a flashback of my own experience.

I met Dr. Deng almost 13 years ago when I suddenly succumbed to a catastrophic illness and became critically ill. Two other hospitals had done their level best for me but I was dying, one life-threatening event after another. From my bed, I watched my family's hearts break as it became increasingly clear that I would likely die before anyone knew what was wrong with me. One hospital was hands on, gave me everything they had, until they realized I needed more specialized care. As for the other hospital, while the staff did their best, I had the impression that they just didn't want me to die with my blood on their hands. What bothered me most was dying without feeling that the healthcare system knew me, or cared about me, as a separate living valuable human being.

Upon admission to the renowned New York hospital of last hope following another near death experience, I met Dr. Deng as I was transferred from the stretcher to my bed in the CCU. It is so difficult, even now so many years later, to accurately describe the encounter, especially considering how sick I was. Suffice to say that I was profoundly impacted by this doctor who communicated with few words, direct eye contact, therapeutic touch, pointed questions, and honest impressions. He affirmed me and in doing so, affirmed my will to fight to live. Dr. Deng was practicing his Relational*Act* theory with great success for decades before he and Dr. Raia initiated research to identify the elements in a healthcare provider and patient encounter that lead to patient affirmation where possible and power in decision-making where it is not. We, his patients, encouraged him to share his insights with others for the benefit of all.

The book is powerfully, insightfully, and sensitively written. The examples of actual patient situations encompass all the drama, knife-edge emotions of all parties participating in the moment as the authors collectively, carefully and skillfully teach the reader what the Relational*Act* is and why it is important in this high-tech modern healthcare world.

I especially love the way the authors have woven Dante's poem into the critical cardiac situations, metaphorically illustrating that only through recognizing each other's personhood can we as patients survive the system, much less the illness. And this is the most important point, without recognition of our personhood, we as patients simply do not have the desire to fight the disease. We must feel loved, cared for, respected, heard, and honored in order to gather our internal resources to get well.

As an old CCU nurse, as a heart failure and transplant patient, as the observer of my family and my caregivers in crisis and in concert caring for me, and finally as a friend of both authors, this book is a clear description of the Relational*Act*, with thoughtfully executed research; it is eloquently written, skillfully annotated and crafted to reference ancient literature; the cover is beautifully designed, it is very well done, very well done indeed. The sum of parts from its co-authors is certainly greater than the whole.

I would recommend this book to anyone who interacts with the healthcare system, which is everyone on all sides of the illness or prevention equation, and everything in between. It is at the same time surprising while familiar, simple while deeply complex; readers will find it challenging and thought-provoking but most of all affirming and hopeful. It is reassuring that Drs. Deng and Raia have made a quantum leap through their research in setting the standard of what exactly we as patients should expect from the healthcare providers who care for us.

Candace Moose
April 06, 2014

REFERENCES

Adigopula, S., Vivo, R. P., DePasquale, E. C., Nsair, A., & Deng, M. C. (2014). Management of ACCF/AHA stage C heart failure. *Cardiology Clinics, 32*(1), 73–93.

Allen, L. A., Stevenson, L. W., Grady, K. L., Goldstein, N. E., Matlock, D. D., Arnold, R. M., & Spertus, J. A. (2012). Decision making in advanced heart failure: a scientific statement from the American Heart Association. *Circulation, 125*(15), 1928–1952. doi: 10.1161/CIR.0b013e31824f2173.

Bourdieu, P. (1977). *Outline of a Theory of Practice* (Vol. 16). Cambridge, UK: Cambridge University Press.

Broom, A., & Kirby, E. (2013). The end of life and the family: hospice patients' views on dying as relational. *Sociology of Health and Illness, 35*(4), 499–513. doi: 10.1111/J.1467-9566.2012.01497.X.

Buber, M. (2013). *I and Thou*: eBookIt.com Store.

Bury, M. (1982). Chronic illness as biographical disruption. *Sociology of Health and Illness, 4*(2), 167–182.

Cambon, G. (1970). Synaesthesia in the Divine Comedy. *Dante Studies, with the Annual Report of the Dante Society*, 1–16.

Carstensen, L. L. (2006). The influence of a sense of time on human development. *Science, 312*(5782), 1913–1915.

Charles, C., Gafni, A., & Whelan, T. (1997). Shared decision-making in the medical encounter: what does it mean? (or it takes at least two to tango). *Social Science and Medicine, 44*(5), 681–692.

Charmaz, K. (1995). The body, identity, and self: adapting to impairment. *Sociological Quarterly, 36*(4), 657–680. doi: 10.1111/J.1533-8525.1995.Tb00459.X.

Charon, R. (2001). Narrative medicine: a model for empathy, reflection, profession, and trust. [Research Support, Non-U.S. Gov't]. *Journal of the American Medical Association, 286*(15), 1897–1902.

Chattoo, S., & Atkin, K. M. (2009). Extending specialist palliative care to people with heart failure: semantic, historical and practical limitations to policy guidelines. *Social Science and Medicine, 69*(2), 147–153. doi: 10.1016/j.socscimed.2009.02.025.

Crespo-Leiro, M., Schulz, U., Vanhaecke, J., Zuckermann, A., Bara, C., Mohacsi, P., & Parameshwar, J. (2009). 473: Inter-observer variability in the interpretation of cardiac biopsies remains a challenge: results of the Cardiac Allograft Rejection Gene Expression Observational (CARGO) II study. *The Journal of Heart and Lung Transplantation, 28*(2), S230.

Cubbon, R. M., Gale, C. P., Kearney, L. C., Schechter, C. B., Brooksby, W. P., Nolan, . . . J., & Kearney, M. T. (2011). Changing characteristics and mode of death associated with chronic heart failure caused by left ventricular systolic dysfunction: a study across therapeutic eras. *Circulation: Heart Failure, 4*(4), 396–403.

Deng, C. M. (2010). Heart Transplantation. In H.-F. Tse, G. Y. Lip & A. Coats (Eds.), *Oxford Desk Reference: Cardiology*. Oxford: Oxford University Press.

Deng, C. M., Elashoff, B., Pham, M. X., Teuteberg, J. J., Kfoury, A. G., Starling, R. C., & Valantine, H. A. (2014). Utility of gene expression profiling score variability to predict clinical events in heart transplant recipients. *Transplantation*.

Deng, M., Cadeiras, M., & Reed, E. F. (2013). The multidimensional perspective of cardiac allograft rejection. *Current Opinion in Organ Transplantation, 18*(5), 569–572. doi: 10.1097/MOT.0b013e3283651a95.

Deng, M., Eisen, H., Mehra, M., Billingham, M., Marboe, C., Berry, G., & Murali, S. (2006). Noninvasive discrimination of rejection in cardiac allograft recipients using gene expression profiling. *American Journal of Transplantation, 6*(1), 150–160.

Deng, M. C., & Naka, Y. (2007). *Mechanical Circulatory Support Therapy in Advanced Heart Failure*. London; Hackensack, NJ: Imperial College Press.

Descartes, R. (1986). *Discourse on Method and Meditations on First Philosophy*. Indiana: Hackett Publishing.

Dreyfus, H. L. (1991). *Being-in-the-world: A Commentary on Heidegger's Being and Time, Division I*. MA: MIT Press.

Dreyfus, H. & Dreyfus, S. E. (2000). *Mind Over Machine*. New York: Simon and Schuster.

Dreyfus, H. L. (2005). Forward to Time and Death: Heidegger's Analysis of Finitude. In C. J. White (Ed.), *Time and Death: Heidegger's Analysis of Finitude* (pp. ix–xxxvii). Burlington, Vermont: Ashgate Publishing Company.

Dy, S. M., & Purnell, T. S. (2012). Key concepts relevant to quality of complex and shared decision-making in health care: A literature review. *Social Science & Medicine, 74*(4), 582–587.

Elden, M., & Levin, M. (1991). Cogenerative Learning: Bringing Participation into Action Research. In W. F. Whyte (Ed.), *Participatory Action Research* (pp. 127–142). California: Sage.

Engel, G. L. (1977). The need for a new medical model: a challenge for biomedicine. *Science, 196*(4286), 129–136.

Elwyn, G., Frosch, D., Volandes, A. E., Edwards, A., & Montori, V. M. (2010). Investing in deliberation: a definition and classification of decision support interventions for people facing difficult health decisions. *Medical Decision Making: An International Journal of the Society for Medical Decision Making, 30*(6), 701–711. doi: 10.1177/0272989X10386231.

Fauci, A. S. (2008). *Harrison's Principles of Internal Medicine* (Vol. 2). NY: McGraw-Hill Medical.

Foucault, M. (1994). *The Birth of the Clinic: An Archaeology of Medical Perception*. New York: Vintage Books.

Freccero, J., & Jacoff, R. (1986). *Dante: The Poetics of Conversion*. Cambridge, MA: Harvard University Press.

Goldstein, N. E., Lampert, R., Bradley, E., Lynn, J., & Krumholz, H. M. (2004). Management of implantable cardioverter defibrillators in end-of-life care. *Annals of Internal Medicine, 141*(11), 835–838.

Gott, M., Small, N., Barnes, S., Payne, S., & Seamark, D. (2008). Older people's views of a good death in heart failure: implications for palliative care provision. *Social Science and Medicine, 67*(7), 1113–1121. doi: 10.1016/j.socscimed.2008.05.024.

Haakana, M. (2001). Laughter as a patient's resource: dealing with delicate aspects of medical interaction. *Text, An Interdisciplinary Journal for the Study of Discourse, 21*(1–2), 187–219.

Harrison, R. P. (1992). *Forests: The Shadow of Civilization.* Chicago: University of Chicago Press.

Healy, K. (2006). Last best gifts. *Altruism and the Market for Human Blood and Organs.* Chicago: University Of Chicago Press.

Heidegger, M. (1927). *Sein und Zeit.* Tübingen: Max Niemayer Verlag. (1962). *Being and Time* (Trans. J. Macquarrie & E. Robinson). New York: Harper.

_____ (2006). *Essere e tempo* (Trans. A. Marini). Mondadori: Milano.

Heritage, J., & Maynard, D. W. (2006). *Communication in Medical Care: Interaction between Primary Care Physicians and Patients* (1st Ed.). Cambridge, UK Cambridge University Press.

Hunt, S. A., Abraham, W. T., Chin, M. H., Feldman, A. M., Francis, G. S., Ganiats, T. G., & Yancy, C. W. (2009). *Circulation, 119*(14), e391–479. doi: 10.1161/CIRCULA-TIONAHA.109.192065.

Jefferson, G. (1989). Preliminary Notes on a Possible Metric which Provides for a Standard Maximum Silence of Approximately One Second in Conversation. In D. Roger & P. Bull (Eds.), *Conversation: An Interdisciplinary Perspective* (pp. 166–196). Clevedon: Multilingual Matters.

King, A. (2000). Thinking with Bourdieu against Bourdieu: A practical critique of the habitus. *Sociological Theory, 18*(3), 417–433.

Krumholz, H. M., Phillips, R. S., Hamel, M. B., Teno, J. M., Bellamy, P., Broste, S. K., & Goldman, L. (1998). Resuscitation preferences among patients with severe congestive heart failure — results from the SUPPORT project. *Circulation, 98*(7), 648–655.

Lanken, P. N., Terry, P. B., DeLisser, H. M., Fahy, B. F., Hansen-Flaschen, J., Heffner, J. E., ... & Yankaskas, J. R. (2008). An official American Thoracic Society clinical policy statement: Palliative care for patients with respiratory diseases and critical illnesses. *American Journal of Respiratory and Critical Care Medicine, 177*(8), 912–927.

Latour, B. (1987). *Science in Action: How to Follow Scientists and Engineers through Society.* Cambridge, MA: Harvard University Press.

Latour, B., & Woolgar, S. (1986). *Laboratory life: The Construction of Scientific Facts.* NJ: Princeton University Press.

Levinas, E. (1979). *Totality and Infinity: An Essay on Exteriority* (Trans. A. Lingis). Pittsburgh, PA: Duquesne University Press.

Low, J., Pattenden, J., Candy, B., Beattie, J. M., & Jones, L. (2011). Palliative care in advanced heart failure: an international review of the perspectives of recipients and health professionals on care provision. *Journal of Cardiac Failure, 17*(3), 231–252. doi: 10.1016/j.cardfail.2010.10.003.

Mackenzie, C. & Stoljar, N. (2000). Introduction: Autonomy refigured. In Mackenzie & Stoljar (Eds.). *Relational Autonomy: Feminist Perspectives on Autonomy, Agency and the Social Self* (pp. 3–31). Oxford: Oxford University Press.

Martínez-Sellés, M., Teresa Vidán, M., López-Palop, R., Rexach, L., Sánchez, E., Datino, T., . . . & Bañuelos, C. (2009). End-stage heart disease in the elderly. *Revista Española de Cardiología (English Edition)*, *62*(4), 409–421.

Matlock, D. D., Nowels, C. T., & Bekelman, D. B. (2010). Patient perspectives on decision making in heart failure. [Research Support, Non-U.S. Gov't]. *Journal of Cardiac Failure, 16*(10), 823–826. doi: 10.1016/j.cardfail.2010.06.003.

Mazzotta, G. (1979). *Dante, Poet of the Desert: History and Allegory in the Divine Comedy.* Princeton, N.J.: Princeton University Press.

Mazzotta, G. (1993). *Dante's Vision and the Circle of Knowledge.* Princeton, N.J.: Princeton University Press.

Mazzotta, G. (1999). *The New Map of the World: The Poetic Philosophy of Giambattista Vico.* Princeton, N.J.: Princeton University Press.

Mazzotta, G. (Ed.) (2008). *Inferno: A New Verse Translation, Backgrounds and Contexts, Criticism* (Trans. M. Palma). New York: W.W. Norton.

Mol, A. (2002). *The Body Multiple: Ontology in Medical Practice.* Durham: Duke University Press.

Mol, A. (2008). *The Logic of Care: Health and the Problem of Patient Choice.* London; New York: Routledge.

Moose, C. C. (2005). *The Grateful Heart: Diary of a Heart Transplant* (1st Ed.). Cold Spring Harbor, NY: Rosalie Ink Publications.

Morrison, R. S., & Meier, D. E. (2004). Clinical practice. Palliative care. *The New England Journal of Medicine, 350*(25), 2582–2590. doi: 10.1056/NEJMcp035232.

O'Leary, N., Murphy, N. F., O'Loughlin, C., Tiernan, E., & McDonald, K. (2009). A comparative study of the palliative care needs of heart failure and cancer patients. *European Journal of Heart Failure, 11*(4), 406–412. doi: 10.1093/eurjhf/hfp007.

O'Neill, O. (2002). *Autonomy and Trust in Bioethics.* Cambridge; New York: Cambridge University Press.

PalaciosCeña, D., LosaIglesias, M. E., ÁlvarezLópez, C., CachónPérez, M., Reyes, R. A. R., SalvadoresFuentes, P., & FernándezdelasPeñas, C. (2011). Patients, intimate partners and family experiences of implantable cardioverter defibrillators: qualitative systematic review. *Journal of Advanced Nursing, 67*(12), 2537–2550.

Pham, M. X., Teuteberg, J. J., Kfoury, A. G., Starling, R. C., Deng, M. C., Cappola, T. P., & Ewald, G. A. (2010). Gene-expression profiling for rejection surveillance after cardiac transplantation. *New England Journal of Medicine, 362*(20), 1890–1900.

Pierret, J. (2003). The illness experience: state of knowledge and perspectives for research. *Sociology of Health and Illness, 25*, 4–22.

Raia, F., & Deng, M. C. (2011). Playful and mindful interactions in the recursive adaptations of the zone of proximal development: a critical complexity science approach. *Cultural Studies of Science Education, 6*(4), 903–914.

Rier, A. D. (2010). The Patient's Experience of Illness. In C. E. Bird, P. Conrad, A. M. Fremont & S. Timmermans (Eds.), *Handbook of Medical Sociology* (pp. 163–178). Vanderbilt University Press.

Roth, W.-M., & Tobin, K. G. (2004). Co-generative dialoguing and metaloguing: reflexivity of processes and genres. *Forum Qualitative Sozialforschung/Forum: Qualitative Social Research, 5*(3).

Schegloff, E. A. (2007). *Sequence Organization in Interaction: Volume 1: A Primer in Conversation Analysis* (Vol. 1). Cambridge, UK: Cambridge University Press.

Shapin, S. (1996). *The Scientific Revolution*. Chicago, IL: University of Chicago Press.

Silverstein, A. (2007). *Sick Girl*. New York, NY: Grove/Atlantic Press.

Starling, R. C., Pham, M., Valantine, H., Miller, L., Eisen, H., Rodriguez, E. R., McCurry, K. (2006). Molecular testing in the management of cardiac transplant recipients: initial clinical experience. *The Journal of Heart and Lung Transplantation, 25*(12), 1389–1395.

Stewart, M., Brown, J. B., Weston, W. W., McWhinney, I. R., McWilliam, C., & Freeman, T. R. (2003). *Patient-Centered Medicine: Transforming the Clinical Method*. Oxon, UK: Radcliff Medical Press Ltd.

Timmermans, S., & Haas, S. (2008). Towards a sociology of disease. *Sociology of Health and Illness, 30*(5), 659–676. doi: 10.1111/J.1467-9566.2008.01097.X.

Tobin, K. (2009). Tuning into others' voices: radical listening, learning from difference, and escaping oppression. *Cultural Studies of Science Education, 4*(3), 505–511. doi: 10.1007/s11422-009-9218-1.

Tresolini, C., & Pew-Fetzer Task Force. (1994). Health Professions Education and Relationship-Centered Care. San Francisco, California: Pew Health Professions Commission.

Varela, F. G., Maturana, H. R., & Uribe, R. (1974). Autopoiesis: the organization of living systems, its characterization and a model. *Biosystems, 5*(4), 187–196.

Venter, J. C., Adams, M. D., Myers, E. W., Li, P. W., Mural, R. J., Sutton, G. G., & Holt, R. A. (2001). The sequence of the human genome. *Science, 291*(5507), 1304–1351.

von Haehling, S., & Anker, S. D. (2013). Cachexia vs obesity: where is the real unmet clinical need? *Journal of Cachexia, Sarcopenia and Muscle, 4*(4), 245–246. doi: 10.1007/s13539-013-0124-8.

von Weizsaecker, V. (1950). *Der Gestaltkreis*. Stuttgart: Thieme Verlag.

Webb, H. (2010). *The Medieval Heart*. New Haven: Yale University Press.

Winnicott, D. W. (1960). The theory of the parent-infant relationship. *International Journal of Psychoanalysis, 41*(6), 585–595.

Wirtz, V., Cribb, A., & Barber, N. (2006). Patient-doctor decision-making about treatment within the consultation — a critical analysis of models. *Social Science and Medicine, 62*(1), 116–124. doi: 10.1016/J.Socscimed.2005.05.017.

Zimmermann, C. (2007). Death denial: obstacle or instrument for palliative care? An analysis of clinical literature. *Sociology of Health and Illness, 29*(2), 297–314. doi: 10.1111/j.1467-9566.2007.00495.x.

INDEX